Professionalism and Reflection in Veterinary Nursing

Professionalism and Reflection in Veterinary Nursing

Edited by

Sue Badger

Andrea Jeffery
**University of Bristol
UK**

WILEY Blackwell

This edition first published 2022
© 2022 John Wiley & Sons Ltd

The right of Sue Badger and Andrea Jeffery to be identified as the authors of the editorial material in this work has been asserted in accordance with law.

Registered Offices
John Wiley & Sons, Inc., 111 River Street, Hoboken, NJ 07030, USA
John Wiley & Sons Ltd, The Atrium, Southern Gate, Chichester, West Sussex, PO19 8SQ, UK

Editorial Office
John Wiley & Sons Ltd, The Atrium, Southern Gate, Chichester, West Sussex, PO19 8SQ, UK

For details of our global editorial offices, customer services, and more information about Wiley products visit us at www.wiley.com.

Wiley also publishes its books in a variety of electronic formats and by print-on-demand. Some content that appears in standard print versions of this book may not be available in other formats.

Library of Congress Cataloging-in-Publication Data applied for

PB ISBN: 9781119664437

Cover Design: Wiley
Cover Image: © Monkey Business Images/Shutterstock

Set in 10/12.5pt SabonLTStd by Straive, Pondicherry, India
Printed and bound by CPI Group (UK) Ltd, Croydon, CR0 4YY

C9781119664437_140722

Contents

Notes on Contributors

Sue Badger MEd Cert Ed RVN
7 Garstons Orchard
Wrington
Bristol BS40 5LZ
UK

**Sarah Batt-Williams MSc Vet Ed, BSc
Hons, FHEA, RVN**
**Senior Teaching Fellow Veterinary
Nursing**
The Royal Veterinary College
Hawkshead Lane
North Mymms
Hatfield
Herts AL9 7TA
UK

**Andrea Jeffery EdD MSc DipAVN
(Surgical) Cert Ed FHEA RVN**
University of Bristol
Bristol Veterinary School
Langford House
Langford
Bristol BS40 5DU
UK

**Rebecca Jones DipAVN (Surgical)
RVN**
Clinical Governance Manager
Langford Vets Small Animal
Hospital
Langford House
Langford
Bristol BS40 5DU
UK

Kathy Kissick MA Ed, Cert MEd RVN
38 Le Banquage
Alderney
Channel Islands
GY9 3YP

**Jill Macdonald DipAVN (Surgical)
FHEA RVN**
Walnut Lodge
Farm Lane
South Littleton
Worcestershire WR11 8TL
UK

Hamish Morrin MSc FHEA RVN
Teaching Fellow
The Royal Veterinary College
Hawkshead Lane
North Mymms
Hatfield
Hertfordshire AL9 7TA
UK

**Hilary Orpet MSc VetEd, BSc DipAVN
(Surgical) Cert Ed FHEA DipCABT RVN**
Senior Lecturer in Veterinary Nursing
The Royal Veterinary College
Hawkshead Lane
North Mymms
Hatfield
Herts AL9 7TA
UK

**Lyndsay Wade BSc (Hons) MRes PG
Cert VetEd FHEA RVN**
**Teaching Fellow in Veterinary Clinical
Skills**
Clinical Skills Centre
LIVE Building
The Royal Veterinary College
Hawkshead Lane
North Mymms
Hatfield
Hertfordshire AL9 7TA
UK

**Perdi Welsh BSc Hons, PGCertVetEd,
DipAVN (Surgical), FHEA, RVN**
Principal Teaching Fellow
The Royal Veterinary College
Hawkshead Lane
North Mymms
Hatfield
Hertforshire AL9 7TA
UK

**Evie Yon BSc (Hons), PGDipVetEd,
FHEA, RVN**
Veterinary Nursing Teaching Fellow
The Royal Veterinary College
Hawkshead Lane
North Mymms
Hatfield
Hertforshire AL9 7TA
UK

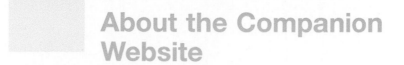

About the Companion Website

This book is accompanied by a companion website.

www.wiley.com/go/badger/professionalism-veterinary-nursing

This website includes:
- Scenarios
- Tasks
- Exercises
- Activities

Introduction

Sue Badger and Andrea Jeffery

This book has been nearly two decades in development, in part because veterinary nursing in the UK has developed exponentially in the last decade and until now it has never been the right time to take a snapshot of the profession with a view to putting its development into context with the objective of looking to the future using the lessons learned from the past. From the 'little green book' that marked the early student days, to the formalised assessment and documentation of veterinary nursing skills within the framework of a professional stance in practice, has been a long journey. In producing this book we have attempted to shine a spotlight on veterinary nursing in the UK in the setting of the last 60 years and to explore aspects of this development that are critical to its future as a profession in its own right. In doing so we have focused on the role of the RVN at this point in time in order to explore the journey from humble beginnings to future possibilities. It is important that we try to identify and embrace what makes veterinary nursing unique and build upon this to develop a clear identity that is accessible to all, and fully understood by the members of our own profession, veterinary colleagues and the general public. It has proven difficult to decide which aspects to concentrate upon, but we have had the support of a number of very knowledgeable and experienced veterinary nurses to whom we owe a significant debt of gratitude. In particular, we are indebted to the contributors who have taken immense care to produce each chapter. In addition, there are others who have played their part in bringing the project to fruition and to whom we also extend our grateful thanks.

It is useful to take a moment to reflect on why, and indeed whether, there is a need for a qualified veterinary nurse in modern-day practice. It can be argued that modern veterinary practice bears very little resemblance to that of half a century ago in that it is far more sophisticated, due to the development of advanced medical and surgical procedures and practices, as well as increased understanding of the psychological needs of veterinary patients as a result of behavioural and physiological research. This has led to increased client expectations as well as the requirement for greater understanding of patient needs, both

Professionalism and Reflection in Veterinary Nursing, First Edition.
Edited by Sue Badger and Andrea Jeffery.
© 2022 John Wiley & Sons Ltd. Published 2022 by John Wiley & Sons Ltd.
Companion website: www.wiley.com/go/badger/professionalism-veterinary-nursing

physical and psychological. A prime example of this would be the major change in thinking, from that of 'a little pain is good in the post-operative orthopaedic patient as it prevents them from putting weight on the affected limb too soon', to 'there is no requirement for a patient to experience excessive pain as a result of surgical intervention'. Indeed the aim should be to prevent this in order to promote healing and maintain high standards of animal welfare. In addition, there is a moral imperative for all veterinary professionals to adhere to this maxim. In this context it can be argued that the role of the veterinary nurse is essential as part of the modern veterinary health care team, not least because of the focus that forms the foundation of veterinary nursing – that of delivering exemplary patient care and welfare by means of informed and compassionate nursing in a professional manner. In other words, today's RVN is expected to adhere to a framework exemplified by the tenet:

Adaptability, Accountability, Advocacy!

Figure 1 provides a more detailed overview of the traits that may be espoused by an RVN in the environment of today's clinical practice as well as the other career pathways that are increasingly being pursued, which include education and training, research and referral nursing.

The training of today's RVN bears little resemblance to the process that a trainee veterinary nursing auxiliary engaged with 50 years ago. At the beginning, training was undertaken by veterinary surgeons as they were deemed to be the best people to train young women (and they were generally 16- or 17-year-old girls at that time) to undertake tasks under their direction. 60 years later, with a few specific exceptions, it would be incomprehensible for anyone other than qualified veterinary nurses to train student veterinary nurses, as the skill set and knowledge-base has broadened and diversified, and this combined with the element of accountability means that that RVNs are no longer considered to be 'handmaidens' or 'a second pair of hands' for veterinary surgeons to instruct in how they would like things to be done as was the case then. Rather, today's RVNs are trained to be semi-autonomous professionals who are expected to uphold high standards and to also hold themselves and others accountable, including their colleagues where necessary. This semi-autonomous status requires a degree of innate flexibility from the individuals that make up the profession, which necessitates a robust training and a requirement to maintain currency combined with a high moral outlook. RCVS registration requires registrants to act in a professional manner at all times and to uphold the highest levels of welfare.

The chapters of this book encompass different aspects of professional veterinary nursing, beginning with an historical perspective to set the scene in terms of where the profession has come from and where it is now in the second decade of the twenty-first century. We have concentrated on what can be described as the professional aspects and aspirations of today's Registered Veterinary Nurse and endeavoured to provide discrete chapters, which cover each of the chosen areas.

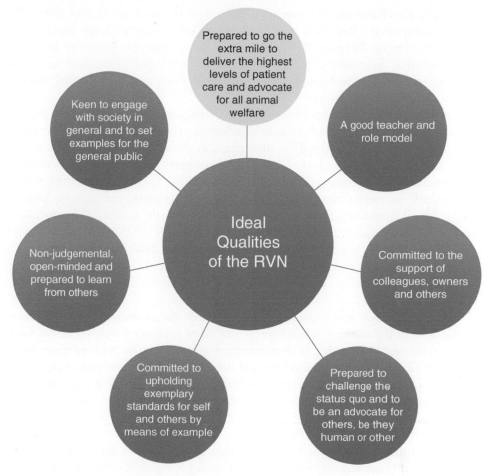

Figure 1   The 'ideal' qualities of a Registered Veterinary Nurse.

As such, the objective has been to produce a book that can either be read from cover to cover by a newcomer to the profession as part of their training, or can be dipped into by more experienced practitioners who have a special interest in one specific area.

One of the most pertinent chapters, 'The Professional Veterinary Nurse', focuses on what it means to be a professional by exploring the development of an explicit identity along with a set of recognised and established behaviours associated with being a veterinary nurse. Within this chapter, the authors have mapped the dates of key events that have been crucial in the shaping of the profession in the UK since 1961. This continues the theme set by the section on historical perspectives, which has been written by an individual who started training in 1970, and so has first-hand experience of the early days. The first veterinary nursing textbook was published in 1966 as *Jones's Animal Nursing*, and was edited by R. S. Pinniger. The second edition, published six years later, contained just two pages on ethical aspects for veterinary nurses, then titled Registered Animal Nursing Auxiliaries

(RANAs). The following entry gives a flavour of the tone set at that time; 'The legal liability of the RANA is that of a servant or employee'. A lot has changed in the intervening 50 years! It would be fair to say that this longevity is a clear indication that veterinary nursing need no longer label itself as an aspiring profession, as it is now a profession with a clearly defined and documented level of accountability and autonomy.

Another aspect of professional identity is engagement with explicit aspects of veterinary nursing jurisdiction as alluded to in another section of the book. The important role that the RVN now plays in the area of clinical accountability and governance is a clear indication of progress on the journey towards a true professional identity. Clinical decision-making is discussed, along with a framework to ensure that, as accountable practitioners, decision-making by RVNs in all areas of professional practice is ethically sound. The process of accountability is also discussed from the perspective of the governing body's response to issues brought to its attention. This is described in detail, along with the potential outcomes that may be implemented in each case as well as a broader discussion of the need to maintain professional oversight in order to uphold standards.

The need for clear and focused leadership within the profession is also discussed in the light of the increase in the representation of veterinary nursing in the wider political context. Leadership is often assumed to be the province of the more senior members of a profession, and whilst this may a reasonable assumption, given the need to bring a degree of experience to the equation, it is also important to ensure that the enthusiasm of youth is not overlooked. Included in the chapter is a discussion of the qualities of leadership that are helpful for those who wish to pursue this as part of their career pathway.

Also included in the book is a chapter that covers another area of professional practice, that of clinical advocacy, an area that is perhaps not given the importance that it deserves, in part because it can necessitate very difficult decisions on the part of the professional dealing with the issues that may arise when engaging with the advocate role. Advocacy is directly linked to autonomy, and veterinary patients cannot be part of any decision-making in terms of their care so the RVN can, and should, play a critical role on their and their owners' behalf. Advocacy also encompasses the role played in both the wider professional and global context and this chapter provides plenty of opportunities for the reader to consider how they engage with this professional and moral aspect of practice.

As previously mentioned, support of the client is an integral expectation of nursing practice today and consideration is given in the relevant chapter to the professional support that the RVN provides for clients as part of the holistic approach taken by the veterinary team. This includes the need to understand the socio-cultural, socio-economic and other factors that play a part in the decision-making that is undertaken in the relationship with the client. The importance of building supportive relationships in general is discussed at length, and includes the challenges faced and overcome in order to ensure that communication within the veterinary team, as well as with clients, is effective. The chapter also explores the meaning of compliance, adherence and concordance and how important these are for a good client relationship in order to ensure optimal care through all patient life stages. The requirement for the RVN to embrace the idea of professional and personal accountability has been a major step in the development of a professional status. It has necessitated an understanding of the concept of a 'no-blame' or 'just' culture and its importance in the provision of a safe working environment for all, as well as acceptance that the RCVS, as the regulatory body, has a duty to protect all who may be at risk of negligent or unprofessional practice.

One of the earliest considerations for inclusion in this book was the role of the veterinary nurse as an educator. There are already many excellent textbooks available that teach the basics of teaching and learning and this chapter does not seek to replace these. It does, however, start with the fundamental aspects of the subject as it reviews how learning occurs, the factors that influence learning and how the alignment of teaching and learning brings about effective outcomes in terms of education. There is also the inclusion of useful insights on different types of teaching activities that can be employed, not only in the classroom, but in the clinical workplace too. There should be a clear understanding by all involved in the training of veterinary nurses that learning takes place in all areas of professional practice, and ideally there should be a seamless framework of delivery that combines the two elements of theory and skills acquisition. This chapter is both relevant for individuals in a mentoring and training role in clinical practice as well as those in a formal educational setting. In addition, a review of different assessment mechanisms provides a reminder of the diverse options available for utilisation and the importance of matching the assessment to the learning outcome to ensure that the most appropriate type is used, the aim being that focused teaching and assessment empowers the student to move in a logical manner from novice to expert in discrete areas of nursing practice, which are then gradually merged into a fully rounded entity as the individual gains in experience.

Crucial to the training role is the provision of individually tailored support for students in the clinical environment in order that they thrive and succeed. Whilst there is a formal pastoral framework to support this within the academic environment, it can be more problematic to ensure that a consistent level of focused support is provided in the workplace. This important constituent of supportive learning requires careful planning and close communication with the associated learning institution so that the essential practical component of veterinary nurse training provides the positive and stimulating environment that is required in order to facilitate well-trained individuals that are able to fully engage with the practice of nursing, albeit at a novice level in the first instance.

It should also be borne in mind that the learning process does not end upon qualification and the continuum should progress through the stage of inexperienced practitioner, loosely defined as the first year of practice post qualification, and beyond. To that end, the concept of 'preceptorship', an experienced individual who supports the newly qualified nurse, has been introduced with the hope that this will be adopted by the profession as an essential element of support for colleagues within the practice team. This principle has long been accepted in human-centred nursing, where it is described as is the support primarily aimed at 'day one' to 'year one' nurses. However, a preceptor may also formally support veterinary nurses moving into a new area of practice, for example referral nursing. This is an exciting area of development for the profession and one that has not been formally recognised before now.

One trait that is considered to be essential within a professional is the adoption of a non-judgemental perspective. As such, veterinary nurses should be aware of any bias, whether it be conscious or unconscious, and to facilitate greater insight reference has been made to the Harvard University Implicit Associations Test (IAT), which is free to access by all. It is a useful tool for anyone working with colleagues in a team setting, with students or with the public as it facilitates a greater aware- ness of the influence that bias has on human interaction in order that it can be recognised and challenged where necessary.

'The Role of the RVN in Society' is a chapter that was considered essential in order to provide a platform for the discussion of the place that the veterinary nurse holds in today's society, and to consider the responsibilities of the members of the profession, not just to patients and clients but also to society as a whole. An initial definition of what is understood by society, including the factors that influence its development, is followed by consideration of the role of the veterinary nurse in society and how far-reaching our societal role is in the context of the further development of this responsibility in the future. There is now an increased under- standing of the human/animal bond and the importance of pets as part of the modern family unit, which has led to the resultant exponential growth in pet ownership in recent times, most predominantly during the Coronavirus pandemic. The RVN can, and indeed should, play a vital part in the education and support of clients and the general public as a whole, particularly in the important role of ensuring responsible pet ownership across the age range from children to adults. In addition to the human factor, animals also have an important part to play in the make-up of a society, they fulfil a wide variety of roles, and in this context the chapter considers the importance of the relatively new concept of 'One Health' and how it contributes to the existing philosophy of 'Public Health', with relevant examples of current issues in these areas, including the emergence of zoonotic diseases as well as disease prevention across all species. The use of the example of antimicrobial resistance facilitates the reader's understanding of the role of the veterinary nurse in these areas, from both the animal/patient and also from human and environmental perspectives. The inclusion of the Royal College of Nursing framework of the 3Ps – Protection, Prevention and Promotion – along with an understanding of Tannahill's Model of Health Promotion provides an insight into the human health care approach that could be easily adapted for use to support clients and the public in general; as such it could be utilised by the RVN in the development of a greater supporting role. The chapter summary provides a power- ful reminder of the breadth of the veterinary nurse's individual and professional role in society; veterinary nurses are no longer just expected to play a role in animal care, nowadays the remit covers a much broader range of responsibilities.

An absolute requirement for any profession is the inclusion of focused research, which in the case of the RVN results in a constantly evolving approach to nursing practice. One fundamental skill required by any professional practitioner is that of critical thinking as part of the process of clinical reasoning, clinical judgement and decision-making. The relevant chapter in this book reviews the role that evidence-based practice plays in the way that veterinary nursing professionals approach all aspects of their work. This allows for a more structured approach to support decision-making, no matter what the career pathway may be. The research chapter considers the role of the veterinary nurse as a clinical researcher using the RCVS Knowledge (2021) five-step process as a template for evidence-based practice or, as we might prefer to title it, Evidence Based Veterinary Nursing. The authors have set out to demystify a subject that many nursing practitioners view with trepidation and thus avoid, which is unfortunate but understandable. However, it is important to appreciate that the adoption of a questioning approach to everyday nursing practice is one of the cornerstones of professionalism. Clinical research is described step-by-step in a methodical manner in order to make the process less daunting and in addition, the chapter provides clarity around terminology, which can often be a barrier to engagement. The objective of this chapter is to give veterinary nurses the confidence to engage with what can be a daunting process in an accessible way in order to inform and develop their own practice, as well as that of others if the opportunity arises.

Although this book is largely focused on the profession as it exists within the British Isles, there is a wealth of knowledge and experience in the nursing of veterinary patients across the globe, from the various veterinary technician roles in the USA to veterinary nursing in the Antipodes. Whilst this book explores the UK profession that has existed in a variety of forms for over half a century, reference has been made to the international perspective where the opportunity arises. Although a table of important dates can be found within the chapter on The Professional Veterinary Nurse, a more reflective history of UK veterinary nursing is also included by way of a personal narrative from veterinary nurses who qualified several decades ago. This will enable the reader to gain some insight into the progress undertaken by the profession since its inception.

Reflection is now considered to be an integral element of individual development within a forward thinking profession and the RVN is familiar with the concept by virtue of the embedding of its theory and practice within the student curriculum, as well as the requirement for engagement with reflection as part of CPD to maintain professional currency for qualified practitioners. A chapter on reflection has been included to enable students to engage with theory that is grounded in veterinary nursing; experienced RVNs can also dip into the content to revise their understanding and to explore new techniques that may be applied to the teaching environment within clinical practice. The reflective continuum is explored as part of the discussion of the progress from novice to experienced practitioner discussed by Schön and Benner. Reflective practice is generally seen by most as a positive skill when applied by the student within the learning environment, as well as by the experienced veterinary nurse as a means of gaining greater insight and improving practice. However, it would be disingenuous to accept it as being the 'Holy Grail' and as such the advantages of the process are challenged in the chapter, albeit with an unsurprising outcome.

Modern veterinary practice is often fraught, particularly so in the present climate of a global pandemic. A pressurised environment necessitates a robust approach to the mental health of the individual as well as other members of the practice team. The RCVS surveys undertaken over the last few years have been reviewed within the section on the professional and political context of veterinary nursing. Areas of concern that were raised as leading to increased stress for RVNs and students included poor career progression and a lack of understanding of the significant role that they played within clinical practice. The fact that the title of Veterinary Nurse is not protected was considered an important indicator of the lack of status that veterinary nursing suffered from as a profession. This issue is addressed in part within the section on the RCVS initiative, VN Futures, which is also discussed elsewhere in the book.

Our aim in developing this book was to provide a template for the reader to engage with in order to understand the modern reality of veterinary nursing, predominately in the UK, at the early part of the twenty-first century. The areas that we have chosen to discuss are those that we believe are critical to the progression of veterinary nursing as an autonomous or at least semi-autonomous profession. The very fact that UK veterinary nursing has formally existed for well over half a century means that it now has a 'sense of place' due to the historical perspective acquired by 60 years of existence which has led to an understanding of the reasons for it's development and for the continuation of its role as a major influence in animal/patient welfare. It is to be hoped that this book will provide a means of reflecting on the past in the context of the future journey.

1 The History of Veterinary Nursing in the UK

Sue Badger

Introduction

A historical timeline can be found in Chapter 3. This chapter provides an account of the development of veterinary nursing from its early days and will reflect upon the grass roots experience of veterinary nurses as well as the evolution of the infrastructure that helped structure this development.

Before beginning on a narrative of the history of veterinary nursing in the UK, it is worth placing it in context by examining the foundations of veterinary science and human-centred nursing.

Veterinary Science

Documentation of the husbandry and medical treatment of domesticated animals dates back to the time of Aristotle and Xenophon; and before that to Hammurabi, one of the Babylonian kings.

In the UK, the forerunner of an organised veterinary profession began with the formation and recognition of the Master Marshalls, a trade guild, in 1356. In spite of this formal recognition, the practice of veterinary science fell into disrepute and did not recover its reputation until the eighteenth century when a veterinary college was set up in London under the auspices of a French veterinary surgeon, Charles Vial de St. Bel. This was followed around 40 years later by a college in Edinburgh. By the middle of the nineteenth century, there were approximately 1000 qualified veterinary surgeons in practice.

In 1844 a Royal Charter was granted (BSAVA 1964) which facilitated the formation of the Royal College of Veterinary Surgeons. In the last century, the introduction into law of the 1948 Veterinary Surgeons Act (VSA) further organised the profession, and subsequent amendments have facilitated professional changes that have enabled the profession to maintain currency within the context of the changes in society and advancements in patient care. The most important of these for veterinary nurses was the VSA amendment of 1966, which considered the prohibitions

Professionalism and Reflection in Veterinary Nursing, First Edition.
Edited by Sue Badger and Andrea Jeffery.
© 2022 John Wiley & Sons Ltd. Published 2022 by John Wiley & Sons Ltd.
Companion website: www.wiley.com/go/badger/professionalism-veterinary-nursing

relating to the practice of veterinary medicine and surgery by anyone other than members of the Royal College. This included qualified veterinary nurses, then called Registered Animal Nursing Auxiliaries, as they were perceived to be 'lay staff' (Turner 1986), in other words their main function was to follow direction given by the veterinary surgeon rather than act as semi-autonomous professionals in their own right.

Human-Focused Nursing

The nurse carer role has existed for hundreds of years but has only been formalised as a recognised profession within the last two centuries. Since medieval times, nursing has formed one aspect of the care of others delivered by religious communities, in particular by the various orders of nuns. It is perhaps unsurprising that war has acted as a catalyst for significant development in nursing care, just as it has for medical specialisms such as the treatment and management of burns, spinal injury, orthopaedics and mental health care, and their associated specialised nursing care.

In the general community, basic care was the province of women from a lower stratum of society, although men have undertaken what have been viewed as caring roles from the beginning of the development of the nursing profession. Before the building of regional hospitals, patients were usually nursed at home by their female relatives under the direction of the doctor, and if additional care was required, it generally took place in a nursing home. It was not until the middle of the nineteenth century that any real thought was given to the need to formally educate and train nurses. The major catalyst for this was Florence Nightingale, who was asked to visit the injured soldiers fighting in the Crimea, and as a result of what she saw, took steps to initiate a formal approach to nursing care. Before she started her work, more soldiers died in the British hospitals than were killed on the battlefield. She reversed this trend by virtue of the institution of a regime of cleanliness, both of the patient and the environment, as well as good nutrition and attention to the individual patient's needs. Principles that we all embrace for our veterinary patients today! Her elevated social status and the work of other notable figures of the time such as Mary Seacole, opened the gates of opportunity to women across the social spectrum who decided that nursing was a desirable vocation to embrace. Florence Nightingale's seminal book, *Notes on Nursing*, was first published in 1860 and is still in print. It makes for interesting reading as, although the writing style is of its time, the general principles of nursing care that are recognised today were documented, albeit over 150 years ago. Chapter 3 of the book is titled 'Petty Management', a title that is unfamiliar to the modern veterinary and human-centred nurse. However, the content is recognisable in that it deals with the need for good communication and continuity of care. The sea change she brought about is viewed as important but ancient history with the passage of time, but it was a seismic event and one of its consequences was the development of the Florence

Nightingale School of Nursing, which opened at Thomas' Hospital in London to teach nursing and midwifery skills. The hospital still contains a nursing museum, which is well worth a visit.

The British Nurse's Association was formed in 1887, with its main objective being to promote the formal registration of qualified nurses. This was followed by the formation of the Royal College of Nursing in 1916 with approximately 30 members. It was notable that this was during World War One as, once again, the requirement to employ the skills of trained nursing staff to care for badly injured servicemen was viewed as crucially important. This was demonstrated by the formation of the Queen Alexandra Imperial Medical Nursing Service in 1902; these nurses were generally referred to as QAs. By the end of WW1 there were well over 10,000 QAs, of whom 300 had lost their lives during war service. The nursing corps still exists today although it is now the Queen Alexandra's Royal Army Nursing Corps. Its members have seen active service in all of the major combat zones including Afghanistan most recently.

In 1940, the SRN (State Registered Nurse) qualification was formally recognised and it was this training scheme that was used as the template for the first UK veterinary nursing training scheme two decades later. The SRN qualification was superseded in 1983 by a new professional register with four pathways, based on the RGN (Registered General Nurse) qualification (Gail Thomas 2016). Three years later Project 2000 laid the groundwork for the move from training nurses primarily in hospital-based schools of nursing to academic institutions. This came to fruition in 2009 when all nurse training courses in the UK became degree-level, a move that was met with disquiet by many who felt that the focus on academic ability at the expense of practical experience would pose potential issues for the profession and the care of patients. However, the ability to develop focused nursing research that informs future practice is undoubtedly one of the important cornerstones of true professional status and, as such, this was an inevitable move, just as it has been on a smaller level for veterinary nursing.

Veterinary Nursing

The first RANA (Registered Animal Nursing Auxiliary), Pamela Pitcher, qualified in 1963 and commented in an article written to celebrate the Silver Jubilee of the BVNA that at the inception of the training scheme a significant number of veterinary surgeons viewed the idea of qualified veterinary nurses with great suspicion! Pamela quoted one as saying that the RCVS had 'created a Frankenstein and would rue the day!' Today, however, the RCVS as well as the veterinary associations now work closely with the BVNA as the representative association of the veterinary nursing profession.

A list of early supporters of veterinary nursing and the then British Animal Nursing Auxiliary Association (BANAA) included a number of very enlightened veterinary surgeons and notable individuals such as Trevor Turner, Oliphant Jackson and John Hodgman as well as Alastair Porter, who as Registrar of the RCVS helped to define a constitution and facilitate the election of the first BANAA Council.

There are clear parallels between the development of veterinary nursing and human nursing, for example, when the one-day meeting to discuss the ANA (Animal Nursing Auxiliary) scheme took place at the RCVS in October 1975, 48 vets and 17 RANAs and students participated. Themes revolved around recruitment, in-practice training and the role of colleges in the teaching of underpinning knowledge. Several training centre principals took part and the consensus was that the theoretical teaching was generally too advanced for the training, as they needed 'girls' who could follow instruction, not 'mini-vets'. Indeed one commented that he supported the training scheme but found no real difference between a RANA and a 'girl' that he had trained himself, indeed overtraining often led to dissatisfaction for many RANAs due to the lack of career progression. The Green Book was applauded as a useful assessment tool but the Preliminary and Final examinations needed an overhaul, as some questions were difficult even for vets to answer! Discussion of the entry requirements led to the subject of perceived over-qualification with respect to the number of O Levels that should be required for entry to the training scheme. Some felt that three or four should be sufficient, whilst one RANA commented that in her experience of training, the pass rate of entrants in this category was only about 30% whilst students with seven or eight O Levels performed far better. Salary was a major consideration, with one vet suggesting that the RCVS were wrong in advertising that this would be around £5 a week for first-year trainees, as his experience was that this should be £15/18 for trainees and £33/39 for qualified nurses. However, a member of the BVNA responded that a recent survey conducted by that organisation demonstrated that some trainees did indeed earn as little as £5/week. Wastage was also an issue according to the employers, with one commenting that turnover was always high amongst women as their working life was only about 30% of a man's; presumably due to marriage and raising children. Hard to believe that this comment was made in 1975; however, there is a footnote associated with this entry to the effect that 'this was disputed'.

The Reality of Being a Veterinary Nurse 50 Years Ago – A Short Narrative

Doreen Lawrence, a veterinary nurse who qualified in 1973, described her experience as a veterinary nurse in the 1970s, and the experiences that she described were perhaps not for the faint-hearted (Lawrence 2020). As a student nurse it could be said from today's perspective that she worked in a toxic environment; her training practice consisted of five male vets, female vets were in the minority 50 years ago, and male veterinary nurses were non-existent. One of the vets was very impatient and thought nothing of throwing instruments at the nurses when things were not going right, whilst the senior partner would happily chat to a colleague whilst the latter performed surgical procedures on patients anaesthetised with ether – an anaesthetic that was still in usage in the 1970s. Unfortunately he was a heavy smoker and thought nothing of indulging in this practice whilst in close proximity to this volatile gas.

Doreen attended the only residential veterinary nursing course at the time, namely the two-term course at the then Berkshire College of Agriculture (referred to as BCA) near Maidenhead. Term one covered what was known as the Preliminary ('Prelim') syllabus and term two covered the Final syllabus

When she qualified, Doreen moved to a one-man practice. There were no hospitalisation facilities, cats spent the post-operative period in baskets, and dogs were placed on a blanket on the floor. Needles and syringes were sterilised and reused – the tips of the former were checked and were disposed of once they had developed a barb. Glass syringes were stored in disinfectant. Dogs were fitted with adapted household buckets to prevent wound interference after surgery, the thermo-cautery with cutting head attached was used to remove the handle and the base of the bucket, then the round cautery head was used to burn equally spaced holes around the base through which loops of bandage or similar material were inserted. Smaller dogs and cats were not exempt, as the veterinary nurse would choose a plastic flowerpot of appropriate size and set to with the cautery in the same fashion. My own memories of this process were that it was surprisingly satisfying!

Doreen tells us that she earned six pounds 10 shillings (£6.50) a week when she started as a trainee at 15 and was able to take the grand total of 2 weeks' holiday per annum. When she left practice in 1977 to get married, she was earning £15 a week. Her primary reason for leaving was that she could not afford to buy a property, as her salary was insufficient to qualify for a mortgage.

I qualified as a RANA in 1976 having also attended BCA, and worked in a variety of veterinary practices including mixed, equine and small animal for nearly 20 years before moving to education and training roles. Mixed practice was refreshing to say the least; some of the tasks that James Herriot was acquainted with were still familiar to RANA's in the 70s. Sterilising the instruments in the cow caesarean kit was one of them, along with mixing up various concoctions and decanting these into a variety of different bottles from 50 to 500 ml, clear or brown, plain or fluted. Dispensing medications was far more varied than today and potentially more risky, given some of the ingredients that were used before Health and Safety legislation was fully introduced. Doreen's reference to the use of Immobilon is a reminder that both S/A and L/A Immobilon were used on a regular basis in those days and although the risks were known, they were not paramount in a practitioner's thoughts.

Farm visits were infrequent for nursing staff and consisted mainly of helping with tuberculin testing by means of documenting cattle i/d and readings, colt castrations and cow caesars. Suitable clothing was not an option other than a pair of wellies and a coat if the weather was inclement; I have many memories of farm visits in the cold and wet, or even snow at some remote farm, wearing boots and a coat over my nurse's dress!

The choice of prophylactic and therapeutic treatments was fairly limited in comparison to today, with a much smaller range of antibiotics, many of which were based on penicillin. Small animal anthelmintic treatment was also less sophisticated; for example, the go-to drug for roundworms was piperazine whilst treatment for ectoparasites involved the use of products like Nuvan Top, which contained organophosphate and was delivered via aerosol spray. Its use generally proved to be a testing time for both owner and cat alike when it came to treatment. The cat-friendly principles introduced by International Cat Care were very much a thing of the future and veterinary pain management in general was the province of a few far-sighted vets supported by input from their equally far-sighted nurses.

Small animal practice was far less sophisticated than today, orthopaedic surgery was limited to the use of implants such as intramedullary and Rush pins, a small selection of plates, which included the Sherman and Venable designs, and stainless steel wire.

Anaesthesia was facilitated by means of induction with thiopentone, later replaced with propofol in dogs and Saffan in cats. Maintenance agents were ether, although this was rapidly disappearing from common use, and halothane, which was widely used, albeit with basic scavenging. What is now considered routine monitoring of anaesthesia was not generally undertaken in general practice, and even the need to maintain body temperature in the anaesthetised patient was generally given minimal consideration.

Nursing management of inpatients was far less sophisticated than today, nutritional care was based on the use of foods that tempted the inappetent patient rather than food tailored to its nutritional needs. Cats and dogs were often hospitalised in the same area – if hospitalisation facilities actually existed.

Clients took their pet to the practice or called the vet to their horse or farm because they were employing the services of a qualified professional first and foremost, as such, they were unlikely to question the advice provide just as they would not have queried their own doctor. Professional status was viewed more highly than today when clients have access to other sources of information, thanks in part to Dr Google! Pet insurance was virtually unknown and veterinary practices were independent businesses, as corporatisation had not reached the veterinary professional at that time.

Veterinary nurses were expected to manage all aspects of the running of the practice from reception work to general cleaning as well as nursing. It's fair to say that the delivery of nursing care was more superficial that it is today, as would be expected as veterinary nursing was still in its infancy. Very little behavioural research had been undertaken and little insight had been gained in the nursing principles that had already been developed and applied in the human nursing field. Patient care was largely based on the medical model and the implementation of an evidence-base was unheard of which led to a largely anecdotal approach to nursing. As RANA training took place largely within the trainee's practice with perhaps 25% of the two-year training period being spent at college, there was little opportunity to learn from other nurses outside the veterinary practice and as a result, some nursing practices continued, as they were considered the norm and were never challenged.

The lack of a professional register for veterinary nurses in the UK was also a barrier to the development of a more professional approach to practice encompassed by a distinct professional identity. But, for RANAs in the sixties and seventies, this was not even an aspiration.

Introduction and Development of a Representative Organisation

Soon after the introduction of the training scheme, it was felt that a representative organisation was required. Although the BVNA assumed its present title at its inauguration in 1965, it was forced to change this to the British Veterinary Nursing Auxiliaries Association (BANAA) the following year due to the fact that the title 'Nurse' was protected by statute. The qualification that we know today was in fact altered to RANA to take this into account and did not revert back to VN until the statute protecting the title 'Nurse' expired.

The Association disseminated information by means of written communication (this was long before the days of electronic communication and social media) and initially a newsletter was produced in-house and posted to the membership. This developed into a journal that included nursing articles as well as association news. A look back at some of the highlights throws up the following facts.

In December 1972 the editorial board took the opportunity to introduce the move from the existing BANAA Newsletter to an association journal which would be published quarterly, and to move production from the existing in-house setup to a publishing company. There was also notification that the proposed first BANAA congress would be delayed until 1974. There were at that time 16 Further Education Colleges that ran part-time ANA courses up and down the country and these were listed in the issue. The BANAA Council Report stated that the ongoing debate regarding uniform was continuing apace, and a large animal committee was being formed to discuss the potential for training in farm animal nursing. The second edition of *Jones's Animal Nursing* was reviewed and the reviewer suggested that the text would continue to play an important role in the training of veterinary nurses – prophetic words indeed.

The BANAA Journal of January 1974 announced two significant events, the first being the change in title to RANA and the second one being the date of the first veterinary nursing congress to be held at the Russell Hotel. I can remember attending this event and was fascinated to hear Professor L. W. Hall relate the importance of monitoring fluid loss and that his nurses collected and weighed diarrhoea to that end!

Moving on to November 1978 we learn from the pages of the journal that London was experiencing a flea epidemic, presumably cat fleas, and that this had made the national news as the *Daily Mail* announced that it was the worst for 25 years, with hospital wards and even areas of the House of Commons having to be fumigated! A report was given of the BANAA Refresher Course that had run at the Centre for European Agricultural Studies, Wye College. The two-day course consisted of lectures from a number of speakers, mainly vets, although two RANAs were also speakers, one on Stock Control and Organisation and the other on Safety in the Practice. The final speaker discussed what he needed from his large animal veterinary nurses, this included the ability to drive, understanding of the farm clients' needs and being alert, as well as the ability to handle farm animals within reason. He also liked them to live locally and have their own hobbies so as not to run the risk of becoming institutionalised.

Finally, the February 1979 journal contained the results of the RCVS debate on a Statutory Register for RANAs. The preamble to this debate stated that discussion of the need for a training scheme was first published in 1955 and at this stage a statutory register with the associated power to remove names for disciplinary reasons was considered to be a necessary part of the proposal. This was rejected by the Privy Council on the grounds that the College could not be given power to control individuals who were not its members. Later, in 1966, the Ministry of Agriculture, Fisheries & Food (MAFF – the precursor to Defra) declined to support giving the College these powers under the 1966 VSA on the grounds that the training scheme had not yet proved itself. At the time of the debate there were around 1200 RANAs and 600 trainees in practice and three full-time (two term) courses in existence.

The recommendations of the Swann Committee (July 1975) would appear to give the opportunity for statutory regulation to be considered again as these included the need for greater flexibility in the employment of veterinary lay staff as well as regulation by means of a statutory instrument which would enable the Royal College to remove individuals from a register on grounds of misconduct. The issue of allowing RANAs to perform certain procedures was viewed with caution as this would require the Royal College to ensure that such increased responsibility was managed and regulated in such as way as to ensure that animal welfare was paramount. On a lighter note, it was reported that the 3rd edition of *Jones's Animal Nursing* was in the pipeline and that it was anticipated that the number of contributing veterinary nurses would increase from two to four.

Present and Future Development

Veterinary nursing in the twenty-first century is a far cry from the account given in the previous section; modern RVN's have a degree of confidence in their ability and a well-defined nursing role which places them at the core of the practice team. The presence of nearly two decades of graduate nurses in the workplace has also contributed to that sense of identity and confidence. Time has moved on from the early days when not everyone supported the continuation of a training scheme. Some warned that a monster of Frankenstein proportions would be unleashed; but the passage of time has demonstrated the necessity for a trained veterinary nurse professional just as the recognition of the need for trained nurses to care for human patients was accepted 150 years ago. No longer are RVNs solely considered as human resources that are part of the fabric of veterinary practice, now they may be business partners and professionals who are able to influence the future not just of veterinary nursing but of a wider professional spectrum, and they also have a role to play in educating society in animal welfare and care. They are expected to adhere to professional ideals and demonstrate these in the training of future veterinary professionals in the context of twenty-first century animal welfare standards.

The cry that first echoed back at the start of the training scheme, that recruitment and retention were problematic, is still a major worry today. Indeed, it is more concerning than ever due to the societal and political changes that have influenced modern life as well as the pressures of a global pandemic and the surge in recently acquired pets. This has led to a significant rise in both workload and stress levels amongst many veterinary professionals and in some cases it has resulted in the questioning of their future within veterinary practice. This is a trend that appears to have been going on for several years as the 2016 RCVS survey of the veterinary nursing profession indicated that there was a significant increase in the number of respondents that were contemplating leaving the profession (25%) in the next five years, with the main challenges identified as client expectations and poor financial reward, along with stress.

Conversely, the survey highlighted that there were positive things about being a RVN including, unsurprisingly, working with animals as well as job satisfaction, with nearly 51% of respondents saying that they would choose veterinary nursing as a career again if given the choice.

One positive change is an increased understanding of these pressures and the acceptance by many workplaces that staff should be able to ask for support when they are struggling. The RCVS Mind Matters Initiative (MMI) is an example of a dedicated support service for the veterinary team. It was launched in 2015 as a response to the rise in mental health issues amongst veterinary professionals and provides an accessible forum for discussion and support, as well as training in the management of mental health issues. A far cry from the 'good old days' when such things were often seen as a sign of weakness, and a welcome sign of a more progressive approach.

The future holds further challenges and, potentially greater opportunities for the veterinary nursing profession in the UK. VN Futures is the joint RCVS/BVNA initiative set up in 2016 with the original brief of identifying the challenges that will need to be faced in the next few decades, as well as the opportunities that the profession must be ready to grasp, if and when they present themselves. The VN Futures interim report of 2016 documented that there were 13,678 veterinary nurses on the Register.

The VN Futures Report of 2021 gives this figure as 20,543. The report also includes a short summary of the 2019 RCVS survey of the VN profession. Nearly

29% of the RVN population responded to the survey and the responses demonstrated that there was a slight increase in diversity whilst the age of qualified veterinary nurses had also increased slightly. Seventy percent of the respondents work full time, with an average age of 35 years, and an increase in the number of part-time RVNs also mirrors the trend towards the more flexible approach to working patterns that is becoming established in UK society as a whole. Most RVNs work in small animal first opinion practice, but 14% work in referral practice, whilst 1.2% describe themselves as practice owners/partners. Although very small, this figure serves to demonstrate the change in status of the veterinary nurse from the 'girl' who was expected to follow direction, to a fully-fledged professional with a well-defined role. Doreen would have found this hard to imagine back in the seventies, as would I!

References

BSAVA (1964). The veterinary profession. *J. Small Anim. Pract.* 5 (2): 195–200. https://doi.org/10.1111/j.1748-5827.1964.tb04237.x.

Gail Thomas, B. (2016). A Brief History of Nursing in the UK. https://memoriesofnursing.uk/wp-content/uploads/A-Brief-History-of-Nursing-in-the-UK.pdf (accessed 24 January 2022).

Lawrence, D. (2020). RANA memories – celebrating 50 years in the nursing profession. *VN Times* 20 (11).

RCVS (1975). Summary of the Proceedings of the One-Day Meeting on the A.N.A. Scheme. 29 November.

Turner, W.T. (1984). The history of animal nursing. *J. Small Anim. Pract.* 25: 307–311. https://doi.org/10.1111/j.1748-5827.1984.tb03394.x.

Veterinary Futures Action Group (2016). VN Futures Report 2016. RCVS.

Veterinary Futures Action Group (2021). VN Futures Report 2021. RCVS.

2 The Professional and Political Context of Veterinary Nursing in the UK

Andrea Jeffery

Introduction

It is important to consider the development of the veterinary nursing profession as one of the starting points of this book. This is in order to understand the progress that has been made over the past decade in terms of the professional practice remit of veterinary nurses. Having an insight into the political players that have influenced and continue to influence that change and development is also important in terms of the context of the chapter. The Royal College of Veterinary Surgeons (RCVS) has been instrumental in driving forward change, and since 2012 there has been a strengthening of position in terms of the title 'Veterinary Nurse'. The 2012 changes to both the veterinary nursing and veterinary surgeons Code of Professional Conduct still state however, that there remain in place restrictions created by the 1966 Veterinary Surgeons Act (VSA), which mean that without parliamentary review of the VSA the title 'Veterinary Nurse' cannot be protected. It is important that the readers of this book understand this as, anecdotally, there have been many calls for changes which are vital but are challenging to achieve because of the mechanisms that are needed for this to happen.

In 2008 the RCVS legislation working party presented to the Government via the Environment, Food and Rural Affairs Committee (House of Commons, EFRAcom 2008) a proposed change to the VSA, part of which was protection of the title 'Veterinary Nurse'. This change to the Act was unfortunately not supported by the British Veterinary Association (BVA), the representative group for the veterinary profession at the time, not because of the amendment regarding veterinary nurses, but because of other aspects of the proposed change. Unfortunately, having considered all the information provided to them, the Government Committee decided not to support the opening up of the VSA at that time. However, having heard the evidence surrounding the protection of title for, and regulation of, veterinary nursing, the Committee understood that change was required for veterinary nurses, but that opening up the VSA was not the way to make this happen in 2008. This is an important point as it shows that there was an understanding of the need

Professionalism and Reflection in Veterinary Nursing, First Edition.
Edited by Sue Badger and Andrea Jeffery.
© 2022 John Wiley & Sons Ltd. Published 2022 by John Wiley & Sons Ltd.
Companion website: www.wiley.com/go/badger/professionalism-veterinary-nursing

for a change in legislation around veterinary nursing which can be used when any further push for legislative change happens. There is, at the time of writing (2020), a consultation with the veterinary and veterinary nursing professions on a proposal for a new Legislative Reform Order (LRO) on the expansion of the role of the veterinary nurse, under Schedule Three of the VSA, and also protection of the title 'Veterinary Nurse', however, even if the consultation indicates a desire to go back to Government, parliamentary time may be difficult to achieve with everything that is happening politically, in terms of Brexit and Covid-19.

The Significance of the Code of Conduct

In 2010 the RCVS veterinary nurses' professional conduct structure was developed, and veterinary nursing Preliminary Investigation and Disciplinary Committees were established. At this time a register of veterinary nurses was established by the RCVS along with the requirements to remain on the Register with a yearly retention fee, a commitment to adhere to the then Guide to Professional Conduct and later the Code of Professional Conduct, and to undertake 15 hours of continuing professional development a year.

Until 2012 someone working in a supermarket one day could the next day be in uniform, wearing a badge carrying the title 'veterinary nurse' and be directed to do something by a veterinary surgeon for which they had no education or training. In 2012 the new RCVS Code of Professional Conduct for both veterinary nurses and veterinary surgeons was published. This was developed by a Code of Professional Conduct working party for veterinary surgeons of which this author was a member, and a further Code of Professional Conduct working party for veterinary nurses. A key outcome in terms of strengthening the protection of the title 'Veterinary Nurse' was a statement built into both Codes of Professional Conduct (RCVS 2012), which stated that veterinary surgeons and veterinary nurses must not hold out others as veterinary nurses unless they are appropriately registered with the RCVS (RCVS 2012). This is an important and significant change meaning that it became a point of misconduct to knowingly refer to someone as a veterinary nurse if they are not.

The Veterinary Nurses Council (VNC) was changed from a committee to a separate Council of the RCVS in 2002, the aim of this change being for the RCVS to align veterinary nurses with veterinary surgeons, who already had an established Council. The chair between 2002 and 2005 was a veterinary surgeon, the rationale being that this was an experienced past president of the veterinary surgeons' (RCVS)Council. However, this was the only time that a veterinary surgeon chaired the VNC and since 2005 the chair of VNC has been a veterinary nurse, thus reflecting the increase in professional identity of veterinary nursing as a profession in its own right in terms of the RCVS as the regulatory body.

The RCVS Council structure and membership, without a LRO, meant that there was no elected veterinary nurse on that Council; the chair of the VNC reported to the RCVS Veterinary Council but did not have the ability to vote or make comment at that forum unless invited to do so and was, therefore, unable to contribute to debate. Part of the membership of the veterinary council at that time was made up of two representatives from each university delivering veterinary education in the UK (one of whom is the head of the veterinary school, the other can be another veterinary surgeon or a lay member). In 2010 the University of Bristol requested that their second representative could be a veterinary nurse who was already an elected member of the VN Council. This was agreed and this RVN therefore became the first veterinary nurse to be appointed to the RCVS Council. This was not an ideal situation as it was not a secure seat because the University of Bristol might at any time have decided that it wished to have a different second representative, meaning that the veterinary nursing voice would be lost.

In September 2015, a Department for Environment, Food and Rural Affairs (Defra) consultation of the veterinary profession took place. This was developed in close liaison with the RCVS through its Governance Review Group (of which this author was a member to provide a veterinary nursing perspective) regarding changing the structure of the RCVS Council and its membership. One of the options proposed for consideration by the profession was to have two appointed veterinary nurses on the RCVS Council. In 2018, a LRO was placed before Government for approval and succeeded. For the first time in the history of the RCVS two veterinary nurses had a seat on the RCVS Veterinary Council and were able to be part of all discussions and vote.

At the time of writing this chapter, there is a further RCVS consultation of both professions across a range of proposals including protection of the title 'Veterinary Nurse' and extending the remit of the RVN under Schedule Three of the VSA (RCVS 2020).

Career Progression and Career Theory

The strengthening of the professional standing of RVNs is one mechanism for veterinary nursing to become a profession with a recognised career structure. This could be similar to that for human-centred nursing in the UK, to include clear roles and responsibilities linked to salary scales and professional development opportunities. This could never be a nationwide initiative due to the business model of veterinary practice in the UK; however, there could be benchmarking across the major employer groups.

The remit of the veterinary nurse is now wide-reaching and covers roles and responsibilities in a significant number of disciplines. When someone transitions from one role to another, it is an important part of the decision-making process, as it is for anyone considering changing their job role or their career direction. This change may be within the veterinary practice where they are employed, a move to a new role in a new practice including the move from primary care to referral, or a complete change from clinical practice into other areas where the RVN qualification can be used. Having a framework to help us make those sorts of decisions is a valuable resource. One such framework was developed by Patton and McMahon (2006, 2014), who developed a Systems Theory Framework (STF) as a way of informing career change. It is helpful as a mechanism for identifying all the factors impacting on an individual who may be considering such a change. The STF, according to Patton and McMahon (2006, 2014), positions itself as a system which considers the interpersonal factors and influences on an individual's career development, such as their personality, ability, and gender.

The STF also considers factors external to the individual that may influence their potential career change decisions such as the current social, political, economic, and environmental influences. When we consider 2020 and the impact that Covid-19, as an external factor, has had in terms of the social and economic impact on our profession, someone who may have been considering moving jobs in 2019 may have decided that the external factors linked to Covid-19 were too great in 2020. Although there is a desire for a career change, they may consider the risks to have been too great in 2020 and therefore delayed the opportunity for change or progression. Using a framework, such as the STF, to support decision-making, enables the individual to make decisions around their future in an holistic way which takes all aspects of their life into consideration.

When illustrating the STF, Patton and McMahon (2006, 2014) use the symbol of a lightning bolt cutting through the framework, as a depiction of how 'chance' plays a part in an individual's career development. Emphasising that career planning and development contain an element of chance in terms of the opportunities which may become available to individuals is important in recognising that there are many factors which influence the career pathway choices individuals make. The message being that change, although unsettling, can bring about growth and development for an individual (McMahon and Watson 2015).

Having ownership of our own careers and the decision-making around the changes we make in them was described by Richardson (2006) as making meaningful the role that work plays in our life and how careers are managed as part of life. Recognising that the factors that influence other parts of our lives can also directly or indirectly influence career choices at any stage of our working life. For example, internal factors such as having a child and that child's journey through nursery, primary, secondary, and tertiary education will impact on whether an individual will relocate as part of their career development. An external influence might be the change of a direct line manager or owner of the business, which means that the ethos of the workplace no longer fits with our own, and so influencing the decision for change. Having someone to talk to about career challenges is helpful and although there are not specific careers counsellors within the veterinary nursing profession, having someone in a formal or informal role at an organisational, practice, or individual level could help bring about a positive cultural change and thus be a possible mechanism to improve retention within the profession.

Careers counselling would be a valuable service to offer veterinary professionals, including veterinary nurses, in particular, within major employer groups. These groups offer career development opportunities to individuals across a large geographical area, enabling movement of staff across the UK and Europe, and this could be a positive mechanism for individual career development. Having someone as a careers counsellor who can support individuals in their decision-making around their career development would be beneficial in terms of retention of nurses within the profession.

If we consider in more detail how careers counselling works, Herr (1997) described it as having five component parts. Firstly, building an understanding of how someone interacts with the external environment they are in and their experience with that. Secondly, as suggested by the term 'counselling', it is not a single intervention that is needed but a range of different interventions. Thirdly, careers counselling is for all stages of an individual's career and should be iterative in its approach. Fourthly, Herr (1997) is clear that careers counselling helps an individual to identify and address professional and emotional behaviours in themselves and others, which may be linked to a career challenge. Finally, it should be viewed as an ongoing process not just an early careers intervention. This ongoing and holistic approach to career counselling was also recognised as important by McMahon and Watson (2015), but is something that is currently missing as a formalised service in the veterinary industry which could bring huge benefit to our profession. However, it could be developed in a less formalised way through the use of mentors or coaches within our practices or though access to advice from the veterinary nursing representative and regulatory bodies.

Our profession has made great strides in recent years to develop careers pathways in veterinary nursing and raising awareness with current students is one opportunity to do this through careers events. These could not only have major employer groups attending to discuss opportunities but also alumni who talk to current students about their careers and how their courses prepared them for their own diverse careers. The British Veterinary Nursing Association (BVNA) with the RCVS have launched VN Futures (www.vnfutures.org.uk/), with one of the work streams focusing on career development. However, more could be done in this space for the veterinary nursing profession in terms of developing career pathways, and the use of careers counsellors could be one way of doing that.

Veterinary Nursing in the Twenty-First Century

In this chapter we have reviewed the 'professionalisation' of veterinary nursing and considered the decision-making around career choices, and this, the final section, considers the views of veterinary nurses in terms of the career that they have chosen. There is currently very little literature exploring the views of veterinary nurses and the profession in which they work, other than the RCVS surveys of the professions. These surveys provide valuable information regarding the veterinary nursing demographic. The first RCVS survey of the veterinary nursing profession was launched in January 2008. At that time there were 7490 veterinary nurses and 3666 student nurses. The response rate was 35% (3869 responses, of whom 790 were students) (RCVS 2008).

RCVS Survey 2008

The results of the 2008 survey identified that most veterinary nurses were female (98%) and white (99%). In terms of their age, 56% were under 30 years old, 31% were in their thirties, and only 13% were 40 and over. The average age was 30, which indicated that as a profession, veterinary nurses were at that time much younger than the veterinary surgeons they worked alongside – the RCVS survey of the veterinary profession (Robinson and Hooker 2006) showed that the average age of veterinary surgeons was 45. This may be expected as prior to the introduction of the first four-year BSc (Hons) in Veterinary Nursing in 1998, the further education training pathway was all that existed and had a training period of 2 years, therefore, veterinary nurses starting their professional training at 18 would be qualified by the time they were 20 years old. The veterinary science programmes within the UK are between 5 and 6 years in length with the option to intercalate, therefore graduates who started their studies at 18 would qualify at 23 years of age at the minimum.

The average basic annual salary (excluding on-call and overtime) of full-time veterinary nurse respondents in the 2008 survey was £17 104, with those who qualified before 1980 earning £21 708 on average. Two thirds (65%) of those who worked overtime were routinely paid for doing so; the remainder either had time off in lieu, with 14% receiving no pay or time off in lieu of overtime.

In the 2008 survey, veterinary nurses were asked to select one of a choice of options in a question regarding intention to leave or stay within the profession. Seventy-three percent of veterinary nurse respondents in 2008 selected the option indicating that they planned to stay in clinical practice for the foreseeable future (the specific length of time was not stipulated); 24% planned to leave within the next 12 months or within the next 5 years; and the remaining 3% indicated that they were intending to leave as soon as possible. Those who planned to leave for reasons other than retirement were asked why they wanted to leave and gave not being rewarded financially and not being valued (30.1%) as the main reasons for leaving. Those planning to leave also stated that they wanted a career change or a new challenge due to the lack of career opportunities in veterinary nursing (20.8%).

Veterinary nurses were also asked for their reactions to a series of 15 attitude statements providing an insight into their opinions and perceptions about their job role and working environment. The responses indicated that while veterinary nurses had high levels of job satisfaction, they found their work stressful and were unhappy about the lack of opportunities for career progression (4.2%) as well as part-time working and the absence of family-friendly policies and work patterns within clinical practice (19.2%).

In the 2008 survey, veterinary nurses aged under 20 years were least likely to say that the role of a veterinary nurse was stressful and most likely to say that veterinary nursing gave them job satisfaction. In addition, younger veterinary nurses selected the 'strongly agree' response to the statement that the veterinary nursing profession offers good opportunities for career progression. However, the fact that they were early career nurses meant that this was not an unexpected response.

Veterinary nurses were also asked whether they would still opt to become a veterinary nurse if they could start their career again. Of those who responded, more than half said yes. Those aged 20 or under were most likely to say they would choose the same career again (75% replied that they would), although these could have been students or newly qualified nurses just starting out on their career pathway. However, this was not clear from the report. Fifty percent of respondents aged 30–39 answered 'yes' to the same question, which was 25% fewer than the younger age group. There was no information available regarding the responses of those older than 39 years.

The veterinary nurses were also asked what brought them the greatest job satisfaction. Sixty-four percent said working with and caring for animals and 33% said that the variety of patients and type of work brought them the greatest job satisfaction. They were also asked what would make veterinary nursing a better profession in which to work. Eighty-one percent responded that better pay would make it a better profession to work in, 36% stated that it would be better recognition for the profession. Twenty-one percent indicated that more respect from veterinary surgeons/employers would make the profession a better one to work in. Better recognition for the profession and pay were also identified as the main challenges facing the veterinary nursing profession at the time of the 2008 survey, along with education and training issues.

RCVS Survey 2010

During January and February 2010, the RCVS again surveyed veterinary surgeons and veterinary nurses registered on the RCVS database using postal and online questionnaires (RCVS 2010). No rationale was provided for why the veterinary nursing profession was being surveyed again within two years of the previous survey. The 2010 survey had a response rate of 37.4% (8829 responses) from veterinary surgeons and a response rate of 31.4% (4106 responses) from veterinary nurses. In terms of gender, 98% of the veterinary nurse respondents were female and only 2% male. The average age of veterinary nurses was 31, similar to the 2008 survey when the average age was 30 years. The average year of qualification was 2003 and almost all qualified in the UK.

According to the 2010 survey results, those who worked in areas other than clinical veterinary practice, and were still using their veterinary nurse qualification in the role, were on average older than those who worked within clinical veterinary practice. The average age of veterinary nurses in full-time employment was nearly 15 years lower than veterinary surgeons, indicating that the veterinary nursing profession was generally a 'younger' profession in 2010 than the veterinary profession, findings similar to those from the 2008 VN survey.

Veterinary nurses working in veterinary-related roles but not in clinical veterinary practice in 2010 had an average basic annual salary of £23260, whereas those working within clinical veterinary practice had an average take-home salary of £16 379. Nearly a quarter said that they planned to leave within five years for reasons other than retirement, with the largest proportion of those intending to leave on the grounds of poor pay. A total of 16% of veterinary nurses in 2010 also had a second job that they did for an additional average of 10 hours per week, suggesting that for those nurses working in clinical veterinary practice their salaries were not a 'living wage' and had to be supplemented with other paid work.

In the 2010 survey, the nurses and veterinary surgeons were asked what the top five best things were about a career in the veterinary profession and there was some commonality in the top five responses, for instance both veterinary surgeons and veterinary nurses most commonly said that variety in their jobs, including working with animals and client relationships, were some of the best things about the job and gave them job satisfaction. However, veterinary surgeons most commonly said that variety in their role was the best thing about their job whereas veterinary nurses said making a difference for their patients was one of the best things about the role.

RCVS Survey 2014

The data from the 2014 survey (RCVS 2014) was analysed in further detail by this author as part of a major research project and the conclusions were drawn from a multivariate statistical analysis. The analysis suggested that none of the following factors were associated with leaving the profession:

- educational level
- age,
- undertaking minor surgical procedures
- amount of continued professional development
- client demands

There was strong evidence that having a second job is associated with an increased likelihood of veterinary nurses leaving the profession. This was also the case with findings that feeling valued and respected by veterinary surgeons, being satisfied with employer support, having good opportunity for career progression, undertaking nursing clinics, and a sense of job satisfaction, if present, meant that veterinary nurses did not intend to leave the profession.

RCVS Survey 2017

In 2017, the RCVS commissioned the Institute for Employment Studies (IES) to carry out a survey of both the veterinary nursing and veterinary professions on Schedule 3 of the 1966 VSA (Robinson et al. 2017). The aim of the survey was to obtain information about three key areas: the level of understanding regarding Schedule 3 and its limitations; how much delegation of Schedule 3 procedures to veterinary nurses already occurs; and the extent to which veterinary nurses and veterinary surgeons would expand the remit of Schedule 3 if given the opportunity. All the veterinary nurses on the RCVS Register at that time (n = 19671) were sent the questionnaire and the response rate was 39.4% (n = 6783). The design of the questionnaire was flawed as the structure of the question regarding what veterinary nurses should be able to do as part of Schedule 3 and the list of response options provided included a large number of skills already legally within the veterinary nurse's remit and the top three listed and selected by both veterinary nurses and veterinary surgeon can already legally be carried out by RVN's under the current legislation.

Despite what this author perceived to be design limitations with the IES survey, the overarching findings were that there was a lack of confidence expressed by both professions in terms of what can and cannot legally be delegated to an RVN, with veterinary surgeons also admitting that they themselves are not keen to delegate. There was an apparent lack of understanding of the RCVS VN Day One Skills and Competencies by veterinary surgeons, which prompted free text comments such as the need for more anaesthesia teaching for veterinary nurses. Significantly, those veterinary nurses who had entered the professional Register via the graduate route had a better understanding of Schedule 3 and delegation than those who had undertaken their training through the further education route.

RCVS Survey 2019

In the 2019 RCVS survey of the profession, there was a 28.8% response rate (n = 4993). For those planning to leave the veterinary nursing profession, the top two reasons for doing so were the same as in 2014 and 2010. These were pay, chosen by 77.3% of those planning to leave, and not feeling rewarded/valued, chosen by 60% of respondents. In addition, 24.8% per cent (compared to 15.4% in 2014 and 22.6% in 2010) plan to leave at some point over the next five years for reasons other than retirement. This is very powerful data as it indicates that regardless of any changes or initiatives that have been implemented to encourage retention within the profession, the actual number of nurses intending to leave within the next five years has risen by 9.4% not decreased; and therefore this is a powerful message in terms of addressing pay structures, career pathways and RVNs feeling valued and rewarded.

The literature review relating to veterinary nursing is based mainly on the RCVS surveys of the profession (RCVS 2008, 2010, 2017, 2019). A key aspect important to note, also apparent in the work by Halter et al. (2017), is that the literature focuses on the intention to leave and does not collect or report feedback from those who have actually left the profession.

Conclusions

The key conclusions are that the factors that predict whether or not veterinary nursing is a career for life are both multifactorial and individual in their nature. Nurses themselves are responsible for ensuring that those they work with are aware of their skill set and that they use their full skill sets within their roles. Age per se is not a factor for staying or leaving. The education route into the profession is not significant in terms of retention, but there are some aspects of the HE curriculum that could be added to the FE curriculum to help build professional resilience in the areas of problem-solving and clinical decision-making.

There is a correlation between being valued and respected by veterinary surgeons. In addition, when veterinary nurses are supported by employers, they are more likely to stay in the profession. Having a clearly defined career structure and mapped progression routes will be helpful not only for veterinary nurses but for the veterinary team as a whole as well as employers. This will enable all concerned to understand the different levels of achievement and required skills to facilitate the teams working more effectively together.

Having a sense of job satisfaction was an important factor in retention. The one area of autonomous practice that might have been linked to job satisfaction was performing minor surgical procedures, but there was very weak evidence that this was associated with the likelihood of planning to leave the profession. Having a second job was strong evidence of intention to leave and pay featured significantly for those interviewees who had left the profession and so pay structure linked to career pathway structures similar to those for human-centred nursing and teaching is an area for further work.

There is the need for veterinary nurses themselves to explicitly express what they need from their roles in order for them to remain engaged. Therefore, being able to share these findings as part of this book and how the chapters that follow will support the continued development of veterinary nurses is important. It is also hoped that the book will encourage the readers to have conversations with others in the profession (RVNs and students alike). It is important that individuals know what their requirements are in terms of their own 'negotiable' and 'non-negotiable' aspects of any role they take. Helping student nurses to identify their own requirements and then seeking a clinical environment that meets those is essential. Encouraging them to have those early conversations with any prospective employer will add transparency to what is expected on both sides. This is empowering veterinary nurses to clearly state the remit of their licence to practice, including the skill sets they have, with their employers and other members of the veterinary team or any other team they are part of in their careers.

Now visit the companion website where you will find additional resources for this chapter: www.wiley.com/go/badger/professionalism-veterinary-nursing.

References

Halter, M., Boiko, O., Pelone, F. et al. (2017). The determinants and consequences of adult nursing staff turnover: a systematic review of systematic reviews. *BMC Health Serv. Res.* 17: 824. https://doi.org/10.1186/s12913-017-2707-0.

Herr, E. (1997). Perspectives on career guidance and counselling in the 21st century. *Educ. Vocat. Guid.* 60: 1–15.

House of Commons, Environment, Food and Rural Affairs Committee (2008). Veterinary Surgeons Act 1966: Sixth Report of Session 2007-08, HC 348. London: The Stationery Office. https://publications.parliament.uk/pa/cm200708/cmselect/cmenvfru/348/348.pdf (accessed 28 July 2018).

McMahon, M. and Watson, M. (2015). *Career Assessment: Qualitative Approaches*. BRILL.

Patton, W. and McMahon, M. (2006). The system theory framework for career development and counseling; connecting theory and practice. *Int. J. Adv. Couns.* 28 (2): 156–166.

Patton, W. and McMahon, M. (2014). *Career Development and Systems Theory: Connecting Theory and Practice*, 3e. Rotterdam: Sense.

Richardson, M. (2006). From career counseling to counseling/psychotherapy and work, jobs, and career. In: *Handbook of Career Counseling Theory and Practice* (ed. M.L. Savickas and B. Walsh), 347–360. Palo Alto, CA: Davies-Black Publishing.

Robinson, D. and Hooker, H. (2006) The UK Veterinary Profession in 2006, London: RCVS. Available at https://www.employment-studies.co.uk/resource/uk-veterinary-profession-2006 (Accessed 28 July 2018).

Robinson, D., Edwards, M., and Williams, M. (2017). *The Future Role of the Veterinary Nurse: 2017 Schedule 3 Survey: A Report for the Royal College of Veterinary Surgeons*. Brighton: Institute for Employment Studies. https://www.employment-studies.co.uk/resource/future-role-veterinary-nurse-2017-schedule-3-survey (accessed 28 July 2018).

Royal College of Veterinary Surgeons (2008). *RCVS Survey of the Veterinary Nursing Profession 2008*. London: RCVS. https://www.rcvs.org.uk/news-and-views/publications/rcvs-survey-of-the-veterinary-nursing-profession-2008 (accessed 10 July 2018).

Royal College of Veterinary Surgeons (2010). *The 2010 RCVS Survey of the UK Veterinary and Veterinary Nursing Professions*. London: RCVS. https://www.rcvs.org.uk/news-and-views/publications/rcvs-survey-of-the-professions-2010 (accessed 10 July 2018).

Royal College of Veterinary Surgeons (2012). *New Codes of Professional Conduct Launched*. London: RCVS. https://www.rcvs.org.uk/news-and-views/news/new-codes-of-professional-conduct-launched (accessed 10 June 2018).

Royal College of Veterinary Surgeons (2014). *The 2014 RCVS Survey of the UK Veterinary Nursing Profession*. London: RCVS. https://www.rcvs.org.uk/news-and-views/publications/rcvs-survey-of-the-veterinary-nurse-profession-2014 (accessed 20 October 2020).

Royal College of Veterinary Surgeons (2017). *Review of Schedule 3*. London: RCVS https://www.rcvs.org.uk/news-and-views/our-consultations/review-of-schedule-3/ (accessed 24 January 2022).

Royal College of Veterinary Surgeons (2019). *The 2019 RCVS Survey of the UK Veterinary Nursing Profession*. London: RCVS. https://www.rcvs.org.uk/news-and-views/publications/the-2019-survey-of-the-veterinary-nursing-profession (accessed 13 December 2020).

Royal College of Veterinary Surgeons (2020). *Legislative Reform Consultation*. London: RCVS https://www.rcvs.org.uk/news-and-views/our-consultations/legislation-working-party-report/ (accessed 24 January 2022).

3 The Professional RVN

Evie Yon, Perdi Welsh, and Hamish Morrin

Introduction

The chapters of this book have embraced all aspects of veterinary nursing professional practice, beginning with a historical perspective to set the scene in terms of where the profession has come from and what it is now in the second decade of the twenty-first century.

To be a 'professional' is a multifaceted and complex responsibility. Working within a profession can give you an identity and a set of recognised and established behaviours and rules to align with. Often, these are considered based upon the individual's role within the profession. For the veterinary profession, we have rules and behaviours specified for RVN's and veterinary surgeons, as defined by the Royal College of Veterinary Surgeons (RCVS) by means of the Code of Professional Conduct for each respectively. Professional veterinary nurses contribute to the integrity of the entire veterinary profession. We often discuss what veterinary nurses should or should not do to maintain this, yet we need to focus on ourselves as individuals, specifically how we govern ourselves in relation to the professional and legal requirements, in addition to personal values and morals.

This chapter will explore the steps individual veterinary nurses can take to meet the brief of a professional.

The Veterinary Nursing Profession

The veterinary nursing profession in the UK did not formally exist before 1961 and has evolved enormously over the past 60 years. Figure 3.1 outlines a brief history of the veterinary nursing profession, identifying key events from 1961 until the present day.

Professionalism and Reflection in Veterinary Nursing, First Edition.
Edited by Sue Badger and Andrea Jeffery.
© 2022 John Wiley & Sons Ltd. Published 2022 by John Wiley & Sons Ltd.
Companion website: www.wiley.com/go/badger/professionalism-veterinary-nursing

1961	The Royal College of Veterinary Surgeons (RCVS) introduced and approved the first Animal Nursing Auxiliary (ANA) training scheme. Those successfully completing the course were called Registered Animal Nursing Auxiliary (RANA) as the title of 'nurse' was protected by legislation and could only be used within the field of human nursing, midwives, and health visitors.
1965	The British Animal Nursing Auxiliaries Association (BANAA) was formed. The British Small Animal Veterinary Association (BSAVA), formed in 1957, played a key role in setting up BANAA and assisted with the running of the organisation. BSAVA and BANAA committee launch an 'official' veterinary nurse uniform
1966	The first book aimed specifically at veterinary nurses was published by BSAVA - Jones's Animal Nursing (1st edition).
1984	A change in legislation released the title of 'nurse' from its protected status (Nurses Acts of 1957 and 1969), and animal nursing auxiliaries became known as veterinary nurses (VNs). Rita Hinton, became the first veterinary nurse President of the BANAA/BVNA.
1988	The RCVS published an 'Objective Syllabus' for the VN training scheme, which helped to define the level and scope of knowledge required by veterinary nurses to help them prepare for examinations
1991	An amendment to Schedule 3 of the Veterinary Surgeons Act (1996) was made which meant that the role of the veterinary nurse became formally recognised in law. A 'list' of veterinary nurses was maintained by the RCVS as part of the requirements of the changes to the VSA.
1992	The first cohort of veterinary nurses qualified with an RCVS approved post registration qualification; the Diploma in Advanced Veterinary Nursing Dip AVN (Surgical). The Dip AVN Medical was introduced in 2000.
1997	The RCVS became accredited as an awarding body for National Vocational Qualifications (NVQs) and VN training and qualification scheme transfers to become NVQ awards.
1998	The Royal Veterinary College, Middlesex University and College of Animal Welfare collaboratively set up the first Bachelor in Science (BSc) in Veterinary Nursing.
2000	The first cohort of Equine Veterinary Nurses (EVNs) qualified.
2002	The RCVS Veterinary Nurses Council was established to discuss policies surrounding veterinary nursing. Veterinary nurses were elected to Council to help drive the 'profession' forwards. Although VN Council can make decisions, any decisions made still have to be ratified by RCVS Council. A further amendment to Schedule 3 of the Veterinary Surgeons Act was made to increase scope for veterinary nurses and to incorporate student veterinary nurses. The first cohort of veterinary nurses gained a BSc (Hons) in Veterinary Nursing.
2007	The non-statutory, voluntary Register of Veterinary Nurses was first introduced and opened. Registration was mandatory for VNs qualifying after 1 January 2003 and veterinary nurses qualifying before this date, who were on the 'list', were given the option to voluntarily register. Those who were registered, became formally accountable, were expected to take responsibility for their actions by making reasoned and un-coerced decisions, and were required to maintain currency by means of regular CPD. At this time, it was agreed that there would be a period of approximately three years between the opening of the Register and the RCVS putting in place a disciplinary mechanism to allow RVN's time to get used to their new rights and responsibilities of being registered.
2009	The RCVS carried out the first audit of veterinary nurse CPD records.
2010	Andrea Jeffery became the first RVN to become a member of the RCVS Council. The RCVS introduced the Level 3 Diploma in Veterinary Nursing.
2011	The RCVS disciplinary system for Registered VNs was implemented on 1st April. A new badge for RVNs introduced which included the words 'Registered Veterinary Nurse'
2012	The Guide to Professional Conduct for Veterinary Nurses underwent major review and relaunched as the Code of Professional Conduct for Veterinary Nurses. The introduction of the declaration made by Registered Veterinary Nurses on professional registration.

Figure 3.1   The history of veterinary nursing. Source: Adaptation from RCVS Knowledge, 2021a.

2013	The first veterinary nursing disciplinary case. A charge was brought against the RVN for disgraceful behaviour in a professional respect and the RVN was struck off the Register.
2015	The Royal Charter closed the 'List' of veterinary nurses and moved all remaining listed VNs onto the Register, making them RVNs. RCVS Council member, Lord Trees submitted a Private Members' Bill to the House of Lords, which would legally protect the title 'veterinary nurse'. The Bill was not drawn and therefore did not get Parliamentary time at this point.
2016	February 2016, an RCVS online petition received over 36,000 signatures. The Government responded to the petition announcing that the title of veterinary nurse would not be given legal protection.
2016	The RCVS Veterinary Nursing Schedule 3 Working Party was established to review DEFRA's suggestion that Schedule 3 of the Veterinary Surgeons Act could be reviewed in order to bolster the veterinary nursing profession. VN Futures project launched as a joint initiative between the RCVS, and BVNA to 'ensure that veterinary nursing is a vibrant, rewarding and sustainable profession – now and into the future'.
2017	The RCVS Legislation Working Party (LWP) established to carry out an overall review of the Veterinary Surgeons Act 1966 and put together recommendations for change to the Department and to Government. Specifically to examine the VSA and make reform, including giving consideration to more comprehensive legislation, which incorporates allied professions including veterinary nurses.
2019	RCVS launch Inspiring Veterinary Leaders campaign as part of the RCVS Leadership initiative which launched the previous year with the aim of showcasing leadership development opportunities for vets and veterinary nurses and highlighting the potential impact on the future of the veterinary profession. RCVS launch new framework for post registration qualifications for veterinary nurses with introduction in Certificates in Advanced Veterinary Nursing (replacing the Dip AVN awards).
2020	RCVS launch Legislative Reform Consultation to gain the public's and the profession's views on the recommendations set out by the RCVS LWP. Recommendations include amongst others, proposals regarding the 'vet-led' team, enhancing the role of the VN, and regulatory processes.

Figure 3.1   (Continued)

Representative and Regulatory Bodies for RVNs

In the UK, veterinary nurses are regulated by the RCVS. However, they are also represented by other organisations. This section of the chapter will explore a few of these, though it should be noted that this list is not exhaustive.

The RCVS as a Regulatory Body

The role of regulatory bodies is to set the requirements of certain professionals, outline restrictions, and set standards in addition to holding the power to enforce compliance. For veterinary nurses, this body is the RCVS.

The RCVS is an example of a self-regulated professional body, responsible for the regulation of the professional conduct of veterinary surgeons and veterinary nurses in the UK in accordance with the Veterinary Surgeons Act 1966. Its aim is to safeguard the interests of the public and animals by ensuring that only those registered with the RCVS can carry out acts of 'veterinary surgery'. The ultimate aim and responsibility of the RCVS is to ensure improved animal health and welfare by setting, upholding, and advancing the educational, ethical, and clinical standards expected of veterinary surgeons and veterinary nurses.

The RCVS was established in 1844 by Royal Charter. A Royal Charter, in this context, grants certain powers to individual organisations or professional bodies to enable them to exercise specific statutory powers. Under its Royal Charter, the RCVS has been given the right to be the governing body of the veterinary profession. Its statutory duties are laid out in the Veterinary Surgeons Act 1966 and it is under this Charter that the RCVS has been able to introduce non-statutory regulation for RVNs.

Title of 'Veterinary Nurse'

The non-statutory register for registered veterinary nurses (RVNs) means the 'Veterinary Nurse' title is not protected, meaning that anyone can call themselves a veterinary nurse if they want to. Many RVNs are keen for this title to become protected, and it is perhaps one of the most pressing aspects of our professional status at the moment.

Changes to the statute to implement full statutory regulation and make 'Veterinary Nurse' a protected title can only be made if there are amendments to the Veterinary Surgeons Act (1966). This is something that requires a change in legislation, which takes time and involves many bureaucratic and legal processes. See the previous chapter for further details.

The RCVS began the campaign to protect the title of veterinary nurse, with a request to Government for a change in the law to protect the title. An official e-petition was launched by the RCVS in an attempt to prevent persons who are not qualified and registered being able to call themselves veterinary nurses. The petition was open for six months from August 2015 to February 2016. Generally, 100 000 signatures are required for a petition to be considered for debate in Parliament (Gov.UK n.d.) and unfortunately at the time, the petition only received over 36 000 signatures. This petition elicited a formal response from the Government, but the title of 'Veterinary Nurse' remains unprotected.

RCVS VN Council continues to put forward the argument and legislation is currently being reviewed through the work of the RCVS and others such as the RCVS Legislative Working Party (LWP) and VN Futures, who are examining ways of strengthening the role of the RVN including further clarification of Schedule 3 of the Veterinary Surgeons Act (1966) with respect to the delegation of acts of veterinary surgery. The LWP was established in early 2017 to carry out an overall review of the Veterinary Surgeons Act 1966 (after more than 50 years of it having achieved Royal Assent) and to put together its recommendations for changes to Defra and to Government in due course. Their mission (terms of reference) include:

- ensuring that the vision for the future of veterinary legislation is given proper consideration
- proposing a list of principles on which any new legislation should be based
- giving consideration to a more comprehensive piece of legislation that could incorporate allied professions and the regulation of veterinary practices.

Feeding into this working group is the RCVS Veterinary Nursing Schedule 3 Working Party, which was established in 2016 to review the Veterinary Surgeons

Act with a particular focus on the role and status of the veterinary nurse. This group's aim has been to:

- determine what amendments to Schedule 3 are possible via secondary legislation
- undertake a survey of the veterinary and veterinary nursing professions to establish a view on Schedule 3 reform
- determine if the College should support further amendments to Schedule 3 to allow RVNs to take on additional tasks
- consider if additional or amended supporting guidance to the Codes of Professional Conduct is needed to aid clarity
- determine if the delegation of certain tasks might be linked to Advanced or Specialist Veterinary Nurse status
- consider the impact across the whole veterinary team of any changes to Schedule 3.

As is apparent here, there are many critical discussions going on at the moment that will lead to decisions being made about the future development of the RVN's professional role and levels of accountability and responsibility.

The Register of Veterinary Nurses

The Register of Veterinary Nurses was first introduced in 2007. At that time, it was agreed that there would be a period of nearly three years between the opening of the Register and the RCVS putting in place a disciplinary mechanism. This period was designed to allow RVNs time to get used to their new rights and the responsibilities of being Registered Veterinary Nurses. It was anticipated that the disciplinary committee would be introduced by the end of 2010. However, it took a little bit longer and was introduced on 1 April 2011.

Until February 2015, the RCVS held two different records of veterinary nurses: the old 'list' and the new 'register'. For those qualifying after 1 January 2003, registration was mandatory; at the time of qualification RVNs were automatically entered onto the RCVS Register for Veterinary Nurses. Veterinary nurses who qualified before this date were entered onto the List and were given the option (and were encouraged) to voluntarily register, and thus move across from the list of VNs onto the Register. By 2015, 86% of eligible veterinary nurses were on the Register and the 2015 Royal Charter closed the list and moved all remaining listed veterinary nurses onto the Register, making them RVNs.

Code of Professional Conduct for Veterinary Nurses

As part of the requirements for professional registration with the RCVS, RVNs must abide by the RCVS Code of Professional Conduct for Veterinary Nurses (CoPCVN). The Code outlines the Principles of Practice which RVNs should use to govern themselves, in addition to defining the professional responsibilities of RVNs, specifically:

1. veterinary nurses and animals
2. veterinary nurses and clients

3. veterinary nurses and the profession
4. veterinary nurses and the veterinary team
5. veterinary nurses and the RCVS
6. veterinary nurses and the public

RVNs must be familiar with the CoPCVN as it provides the foundation for their role in practice.

Strategic Plan

The Strategic Plan is a roadmap set out by the RCVS to facilitate its work towards the vision: 'To be recognised as a trusted, compassionate and proactive regulator, and a supportive and ambitious Royal College, underpinning confident veterinary professionals of whom the UK can be proud' (RCVS 2020a).

The overarching aim is to direct the profession forwards whilst addressing important areas such as learning, leadership, mental health, and global reach and innovation. RVNs should be familiar with this and consider how it affects them and their future practice, especially at a time where there is much discussion around the veterinary nurse profession and the permitted tasks of its members.

Representation for Veterinary Nurses

There are several representative bodies for veterinary nurses, including the British Veterinary Nursing Association (BVNA). The BVNA exists to 'promote animal health and welfare through the ongoing development of professional excellence in veterinary nursing' (BVNA 2021a). It plays an important role as the only representative body for veterinary nurses in the UK. The BVNA was first established in 1965 and since its beginnings has played a significant part in promoting, representing, and advancing the status of veterinary nurses. Crucially, the BVNA supports veterinary nurses and other practice staff, providing access to a free Members Advisory Helpline, managed by professionals providing advice on employment law plus many other issues.

The role of the BVNA extends to:

- representing the veterinary nursing profession and specifically its members
- developing, providing, and monitoring continuing professional development (CPD) for veterinary nurses
- providing education and training for associated individuals and allied professionals
- promoting the veterinary nursing profession and working proactively with other organisations and professions to shape its future development
- disseminating advice and guidance to its members
- offering a Members Advisory Service providing advice on employment law, financial matters, and many other issues.

(BVNA 2021b)

Other representative bodies include VN Futures (to be discussed later on in this chapter) and the Veterinary Defence Society (VDS). The VDS provides insurance to practices against civil claims of negligence in addition to providing support and representation to veterinary surgeons and RVNs throughout RCVS disciplinary procedures. Each member is given criminal and disciplinary cover (https://www.thevds.co.uk/our-policy). In most instances RVNs will be covered directly by their employers. Locum RVNs and those who are working for themselves should either check that they are covered by the practice employing them or obtain individual membership with the VDS.

The Disciplinary Procedure

The disciplinary process is a civil procedure undertaken by the governing body to ensure that those who are registered are conducting themselves according to the professional requirements. This is not a police system, and it should not be feared, as it is undertaken only for those cases that fall below the standard of behaviour expected of an RVN; ultimately, members of the profession can have charges brought against them of professional misconduct. If an individual is found guilty of charges of serious professional misconduct (the wording of the Veterinary Nursing Rules is 'disgraceful conduct in any professional respect') (RCVS 2014), or found unfit to practice because of a criminal conviction, the governing body can remove that member from the register. By publicly stating and determining if a member of the profession has done anything wrong, the public are reassured that the profession is only made up of members who are trustworthy and held in the highest regard.

The RVN Disciplinary Committee is the branch of the RCVS that hears any charges of 'disgraceful conduct in a professional respect' brought against an RVN. There are three stages to an RCVS Disciplinary Procedure. Figure 3.2 outlines these stages.

Whistleblowing

Whistleblowing describes the action of employees raising concerns about wrongdoing they believe to be occurring in the workplace (Welsh and Bayliss 2013). It is generally accepted that professions serving the general public are expected to practise in a way that is transparent, and thus misconduct and malpractice should be reported and handled to protect public interest. Instances of whistleblowing are protected in the Employment Rights Act (1996), as amended under The Public Interest Disclosure Act (1998). This Act protects employees from detrimental treatment from employers if they 'blow the whistle' and applies to all except members of the armed forces, intelligence officers, volunteers, and self-employed persons. Protection is ensured when a qualifying disclosure is made about malpractice. Examples include:

- criminal offences
- failure to comply with legal obligation

Stage One: Assessment and investigation	• RCVS first receive a complaint from a member of the public or colleague (this could be a whistleblowing event from another nurse)
	• A Case Manager is assigned
	• Information is collated, including a written response from the person being investigated, which is shared with the person who raised the concern to check for accuracy
	• Further information may be sought from anyone who may be able to help with the investigation
	• Clinical records may be accessed if necessary
	• At this stage, the RCVS may send their Veterinary Investigators to meet with the RVN and anybody deemed necessary to then report back to the Case Manager
	• Witness statements and expert reports may also be gathered
	• The case will be considered by the Case Examiners Group, (CEG), consisting of the Case Manager, a veterinary Case Examiner and an external, non-veterinary Case Manager.
	• Meetings carried out by the CEG are conducted behind closed doors and neither the RVN, nor the person who raised the concern are able to attend.
	• The CEG will look to see if there is an arguable case that involves a potential breach of professional conduct. If it is deemed that there has been, the CEG will also look to see if it is possible to prove the case – if it is not possible then it could be concluded that there is little point in pursuing it.
	• Actions of the CEG at this point include:
	    Closing the matter (no action)
	    Closing the matter and issuing advice
	    Deciding there is an arguable case and referral to Stage Two, the PIC who will decide whether it will proceed to Stage Three.
	• Decisions by the CEG must be unanimous, otherwise they will be referred to the PIC
	• Cases whereby the findings are considered to be of a potentially serious nature may be directly referred to the PIC
	• The RVN and person who raised the concern will be notified of the decision by the CEG
	
	Throughout Stage One, the Case Manager may seek guidance from the Chairman of the RVN Preliminary Investigation Committee (RVNPIC) or the Head of Professional Conduct (HPC) at the RCVS

Stage Two: RVN Preliminary Investigation Committee	• The PIC considers whether it is a realistic prospect that the RVN's fitness to practice is affected and whether it amounts to serious professional misconduct
	• Similarly to the CEG meetings, the PIC meetings are strictly confidential and are not attended by the RVN or the person who raised the concern
	• The RVN will be asked to provide CPD records from the past three years in addition to confirming indemnity insurance details at this stage
	• Here, the RVNPIC may decide to:
	    Close the case with no further action
	    Close the case and issue advice
	    Hold a case open for up to two years (with or without a follow-up visit by RCVS Veterinary Investigators)
	    Refer a complaint to the RVN Disciplinary Committee (RVNDC) for a hearing. This will only occur if it is deemed there is a realistic prospect of the DC ruling a case of professional misconduct.

Figure 3.2 Disciplinary steps faced by RVNs in cases of disgraceful conduct in a professional respect. Source: Based on RCVS 2021a.

Stage Three: Disciplinary Committee Hearing	• A formal hearing will take place (similar to a court hearing) • Persons involved, including witnesses may be asked to attend to give evidence, under oath. • RVNDC hearings are usually offered within 12 months of the concern against the RVN formally being raised • If the RVN wishes to appeal a decision of suspension or removal from the Register, this will be heard by a senior barrister (Queen's Council)

Figure 3.2   (Continued)

- miscarriages of justice
- threats to an individual's health and safety
- damage to the environment
- a deliberate attempt to cover up the above

(Public Interest Disclosure Act 1998)

As per the Principles of Practice, RVNs work with honesty and integrity, independence and impartiality, to build client trust and maintain appropriate levels of professional accountability, among other responsibilities (RCVS 2021c). These behaviours emphasise that RVNs have a duty to raise concerns of any professional practice that may impede patient care or exploit or undermine the trust of clients. Additionally, due to protection of public interest, RVNs have a moral obligation to voice concerns of malpractice.

The RCVS has no explicit whistleblowing policy; however, it recommends initially trying to resolve the issue internally by discussing the matter with senior personnel. If this is not possible or is deemed inappropriate, the individual wishing to report the issue should raise their concern with the RCVS Professional Conduct Department (RCVS 2020b). There are many situations in which veterinary nurses and student veterinary nurses could potentially witness malpractice or misconduct. It can feel uncomfortable to raise these and many people will try to avoid conflict. Therefore, RVNs must understand and feel confident with how to have difficult conversations in practice.

Anyone who does decide to blow the whistle must do so with honesty and justifiable reasoning, i.e. they need to believe the information to be true and should be able to substantiate it. Furthermore, the context in which the event occurred should be considered; RVNs should be able to recognise and differentiate between genuine mistakes and malpractice. Welsh and Bayliss (2013) suggest that frequent undertaking of clinical audits in addition to completing incident reports when they occur will help with pattern recognition and highlight areas for improvement in addition to highlighting potential malpractice.

It is important to note that workplace harassment is a criminal offence and is unlawful under the Equality Act 2010. Although bullying is not against the law per se, many bullying behaviours pertain to harassment. Harassment is against the law where the unwanted behaviour is related to age, sex, disability, gender reassignment, marriage and/or civil partnership, pregnancy and/or maternity, race, religion, or belief and sexual orientation (Equality Act 2010). If an RVN experiences or witnesses harassment, they should be aware that this is a justifiable whistleblowing situation.

Crowe (2015) defined workplace bullying as offensive, intimidating, malicious, insulting or humiliating behaviour, or an abuse of power or authority over employees, which may cause them to suffer stress. A recent survey (2017) conducted by VetNurse.co.uk and VetSurgeon.org found that of the 677 respondents, 344 (51%) identified that they were on the receiving end of sustained patterns of behaviour, usually from one person, which seemed designed to make their life unpleasant. These findings suggest that bullying may be prevalent and a serious issue within the profession and although not formally investigated as such, these behaviours could indicate an issue with harassment. Whistleblowing in these situations can be imperative in order to improve the well-being of staff and clients.

Ultimately, whistleblowing can result in disciplinary action by the RCVS, or criminal action.

The Autonomous RVN

Accountability and Autonomy

Accountability is one of the key professional standards expected of RVNs. At its most basic, professional accountability means being responsible for one's actions and decisions and accepting the consequences of any actions and decisions made. In practical terms, this means that professionals are expected to abide by a set of rules and 'standards' set out by relevant law and their professional body (usually in the form of a Code of Conduct) and they may be called upon to justify their actions. Not abiding by these rules could lead to formal complaints, which may then lead to disciplinary and legal proceedings. In addition, professionals are also accountable to certain people and in most instances, these groups will be identified in a Code of Conduct.

Achieving a certain level of professional *autonomy* is another feature ascribed to occupations that have achieved professional status. Autonomy is described as the 'capacity to think, make decisions and to take action independently of others' (Mason and Whitehead 2003).

The law (for example, the Veterinary Surgeons Act 1966) and our Code of Professional Conduct are for the most part clear; veterinary nurses are not yet in a position legally or professionally to call themselves autonomous practitioners. Moreover, whilst there are some exceptions to Section 19 of the Veterinary Surgeons Act, which restricts the practice of registered veterinary surgery to veterinary surgeons, a degree of autonomy can sometimes extend to the general public.

A good example of this, under Schedule 3 of the Act, is the Exemptions from Restrictions on Practice of Veterinary Surgery, which allows:

> The rendering in an emergency of first aid for the purpose of saving life or relieving pain or suffering' by 'unqualified persons'
>
> (Veterinary Surgeons Act 1966)

In order to do this, a decision is made that an immediate intervention is necessary in order to save the patient's life or relieve suffering which will involve an assessment of its status. In this context RVNs (and members of the public) are *sometimes* allowed to make autonomous decisions. Many RVNs will act with varying degrees of autonomy in their role every day, and this understanding has worked successfully for RVNs employers, clients, and patients for many years. However, it is important to ensure that you are aware of legal standpoints regarding some of these issues.

In addition to the regulations set out by the Veterinary Nursing Council, veterinary nurses must be aware of the legislation detailing what they are legally allowed to do. The Veterinary Surgeon's Act (1966) explains this, with specific delegation to veterinary nurses in Schedule 3. Veterinary nurses must act within these laws and regulations, in addition to aligning with their individual practice procedures. However, autonomy can enable RVNs to be individuals within a regulated role. Being a professional means decision-making is informed by the remit of the laws and regulations of this role, yet autonomy allows us to make these decisions as individuals because of the acceptance of accountability.

There is progression towards greater autonomy for veterinary nurses. In 2015, a new Supplemental Charter came into operation, recognising for the first time that veterinary nursing is a profession in its own right. The Veterinary Nursing Council, under the bye-laws, set standards and requirements for the education of veterinary nurses, in addition to the standards for professional conduct. The bye-laws also outline the requirement for veterinary nurses to face disciplinary action if they do not meet these standards, or breech professional conduct. However, it is the RCVS Council that decides upon who may enter, be removed from, or reinstated onto the Register of Veterinary Nurses. Ultimately, the veterinary nursing profession is not fully autonomous at this time despite greater responsibility being delegated to veterinary nursing led bodies.

Continuing Professional Development and Lifelong Learning

Autonomy also extends to veterinary nurses' continuing education and development. RVNs are required, not only to undertake a minimum requirement of CPD each year, but also to keep a record of this. The RCVS CoPCVN makes it very clear that all RVNs are obliged to maintain and continue to develop their professional knowledge and skills (CoPcVN 3.3) (RCVS 2021b). CPD is therefore mandatory for all RVNs and should be seen as the continuous development of capability and competence. It is the personal responsibility of all RVNs to undertake and record CPD.

There are no iterated rules defining what subjects veterinary nurses must focus on, and many may be unsure in which areas they should undertake CPD. It is worth considering two aspects; specific areas of interest and how CPD may be used to enhance knowledge and/or skills in the areas of work. Considering personal motivations, for example, professional interests, personal motivational drives in veterinary nursing and preferred aspects of the role, may help to direct you to particular areas of study. Figure 3.3 indicates types of CPD that can be used to contribute to an RVN's record.

Formal	Workplace	Self-directed
Clinical skills lab Conference Course Distance learning (formal/webinar/other) External qualification Seminar Workshop	Case discussion Clinical audit In-house training Peer feedback Significant event analysis Work-based observation	Preparing a new lecture Preparing a paper Research Veterinary reading

Figure 3.3   Acceptable activities to log as CPD within the RCVS 1CPD recording platform. Source: Based on RCVS 2021b.

Ideally, to ensure that a breadth of skills are covered, a range of activities from each category (formal, workplace, and self-directed) should be chosen. The variety of acceptable activities ensures that CPD should be accessible to all veterinary nurses.

From 1 January 2020, the RCVS CPD compliance policy changed to enforce a requirement of 15 hours per year, in contrast to the previously stated minimum of 45 hours across 3 years (RCVS 2019). Further to this change, a new digital recording platform, 1CPD, was launched by the RCVS. It can be accessed via a Smartphone app, or as an online web version. As a component of this change, RVNs are encouraged to reflect upon the CPD activities they have carried out. Reflection is an important aspect, as already discussed, and thus including this to contextualise and improve learning should be seen as fundamental.

CPD can help to maintain and encourage interest in your work by allowing exploration and discovery of new information. Interest in your work is important for many reasons including ensuring diligence, focus, job satisfaction and not least, patient care. Different members of the team will have different interests, and therefore the combination of these should lead to reduced knowledge gaps in the team overall, ultimately meaning there should be no 'gaps' in best practice and high standards of nursing care. If everyone in the team undertakes CPD in a variety of areas, the knowledge base of the team will be broad. Creating opportunities to learn from one another can be hugely beneficial, and enjoyable. These initiatives demonstrate leadership skills, in addition to promoting a learning environment within the workplace. Taking the time to reflect upon what you enjoy and what you want to learn more about could help with career planning and achieving career goals.

By engaging in lifelong learning, RVNs can share their knowledge to inspire and motivate others, nurturing a positive and motivated team. Individuals should seek to share knowledge with others wherever appropriate. These actions may not only raise the profile of the practice with improved knowledge and understanding but can directly influence improved patient care and education.

By taking responsibility for their learning and sharing acquired knowledge and skills, RVNs can routinely demonstrate aspects of leadership, something that has historically been limited to those occupying senior roles. However, all RVNs have a responsibility to use an evidence-based approach to practice in order to deliver high-standards of care in alignment with best practice recommendations. Thus, self-regulation of education through developing interests and skills, in addition to reducing knowledge gaps, all contribute to leadership behaviours.

RVNs as Leaders

At present, RVNs are taking on greater responsibility and practicing specialised skills far more commonly within veterinary practice than they did historically. It is expected that future changes to professional legislation and regulation will see increased levels of RVN responsibility that will require further adaption of the role, leading to the performance of more complex skills and procedures. With this increased responsibility, many RVNs will see themselves rising to positions of leadership, whether that be specialised, advanced, or senior roles. It is perhaps the belief that only those in more senior positions should be 'leaders'; however, it is important that leadership concepts are understood to enable individuals to set and meet personal and practice targets and objectives. Leadership is a complex and dynamic concept, especially in the veterinary nursing profession where roles are changeable and ever-developing. Key leadership behaviours have been identified as power, influence, kindness, intelligence, innovation, charisma, and goal-focus (Curtis et al. 2011). Leadership means different things to different people, and thus there will be variation in its definition. However, identifying personal motivations and goals, working towards them with focus, as well as sharing your experiences and knowledge with others, may help you to establish yourself as a leader. Figure 3.4 shows the key characteristics required for leadership development.

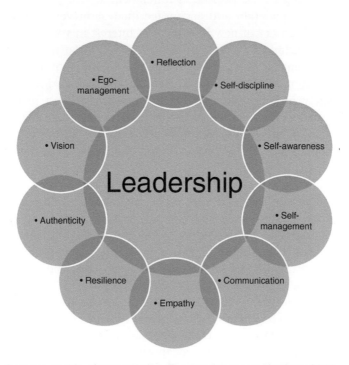

Figure 3.4   Core leadership characteristics. Source: Based on Kerrigan 2018.

Self-assessment of performance of these behaviours contributes to autonomy and professional development. The ability to reflect and learn from experiences and individual performances can lead to improved practice. Empathising with colleagues and understanding how your own mindset can affect your work helps to maintain a professional stance whilst building rapport with the team. Finally, knowing when you are wrong is essential to enable development of the team and improve standards of care by means of reflection and learning.

Personal Values and Professionalism

Personal values can affect clinical judgement and decision-making and thus must be considered when discussing autonomy and accountability. Identifying personal values and the strategies we put in place to follow them will help us to recognise the effect they have on our professional practice. Setting guidelines and boundaries that you are not willing to cross will ensure self-governance. However, RVNs must also consider the consequences of their actions in addition to accountability and should always work within the law and Code of Professional Conduct. As our personal values are important to us, when seeking employment, it is vital to ensure that the practice values align with yours as this may help to avoid any conflict between personal and professional values and protect well-being.

The RVN as a Policymaker

A day in the life of a veterinary nurse will be defined by numerous decisions in relation to client and patient care, and the smooth running of the practice, or ward, depending upon the practice type. According to Fraser (2019), there are two types of decision-making, which are described as system one and system two respectively. System one decisions are made quickly, relying upon instinct and prior experience, whereas system two decisions are systematic, taking into account many influencing factors. In practice, decisions should be made considering the intended outcomes, thus practitioners should be making most, if not all, decisions as system two decisions. To do this, a solid understanding of the evidence base and practice policies is required.

In a world where clients question professionals' decisions and motivations, it is important to adopt a standardised approach to practice. Whilst this is not necessarily possible in all aspects spanning the entire profession, individual veterinary practices can build upon existing evidence-bases, or obtain novel data to set their own benchmarks in order to provide a foundation for policymaking and consistency in patient, client and practice approaches.

Standard operating procedures (SOPs) should be created using a clearly defined decision-making process, utilising a wide evidence-base where possible.

Policymaking can assist decision-making in addition to ensuring quality improvement and best practice standards. To be able to achieve this, the principles of clinical governance must be practised. The RCVS Code of Professional Practice for

Veterinary Nurses states that clinical governance must be undertaken (Section 1.7 CoPCVN) (RCVS 2021c). Clinical governance is the overarching process designed to achieve best practice. It incorporates reflective practice, analysis of outcomes and identification of areas for improvement. Firstly, consideration of clinical effectiveness, in other words how well procedures actually achieve what they are intended to. To accomplish this, clinical audits must be carried out as they can provide the evidence necessary to create a policy. It is a process whereby any member of the practice can raise a question, or area of concern, with a view to improving practice. Figure 3.5 demonstrates how audits can inform change leading towards the goal of improvement in clinical practice.

In veterinary medicine generally, evidence-based practice is thought to be critical to driving advancements in clinical practice. Many areas, however, lack a robust wealth of evidence. Regular clinical auditing can assist practices by analysing data to improve patient care. It must be noted that clinical audits are not research. Although clinical auditing involves the collection and analysis of data, it aims to create knowledge necessary for the improvement of certain areas of practice, whereas research aims to create new knowledge to inform best practice. Research is imperative to the advancement of the veterinary profession. However, auditing allows us to focus on clinically important issues for individual practices, helping to improve standards within the clinical environment. This is advantageous as it encourages targeted and achievable changes, whereas research provides general recommendations across areas that may vary from practice to practice depending upon resources, such as staff and equipment, in addition to caseload and financial considerations. Fundamentally, the use of a clinical audit ethos influences how practices govern themselves by considering evidence, leading to policy creation and improvement.

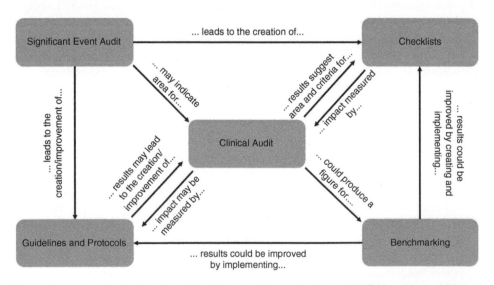

Figure 3.5   Impact of clinical auditing. Source: Adaptation from RCVS Knowledge 2021b.

Clinical governance can be carried out by any member of the veterinary team. Policymaking forms part of clinical governance. Clinical governance is an activity outlined as a specific responsibility of the RVN in the CoPCVN: 'veterinary nurses must ensure that clinical governance forms part of their professional activities' (Section 1.7). As policymaking is within the remit of a veterinary nurse, it is imperative that they understand and can contribute to this practice activity. Creating a policy can be complex and requires collaboration of multiple team members; RVNs can be crucial to this process and thus it is necessary for them to understand the steps involved to promote best practice.

Veterinary nurses have a primary role in promoting the welfare of their patients. Arguably, ensuring best practice is encompassed within this. Thus, in addition to the necessity for participation in clinical governance, veterinary nurses have a responsibility to carry out auditing processes.

The auditing process rarely involves just one member of the team. This may be daunting for less experienced veterinary nurses who are still building upon their skillset, observation, and participation. However, as will become clear, there are many steps involved in the clinical auditing process, enabling opportunity for contribution by individuals with reduced levels of responsibility.

Clinical Auditing: The Process

The first decision to make is which type of clinical audit process should be adopted. Figure 3.6 outlines the differences between the four approaches to clinical audits, namely structure, process, outcome, and significant event.

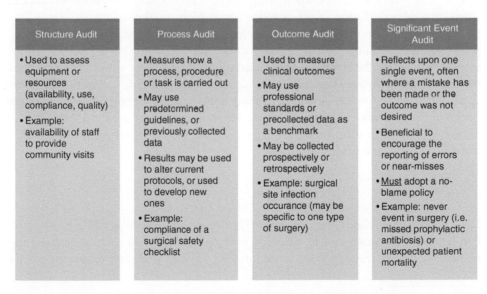

Structure Audit	Process Audit	Outcome Audit	Significant Event Audit
• Used to assess equipment or resources (availability, use, compliance, quality) • Example: availability of staff to provide community visits	• Measures how a process, procedure or task is carried out • May use predetermined guidelines, or previously collected data • Results may be used to alter current protocols, or used to develop new ones • Example: compliance of a surgical safety checklist	• Used to measure clinical outcomes • May use professional standards or precollected data as a benchmark • May be collected prospectively or retrospectively • Example: surgical site infection occurance (may be specific to one type of surgery)	• Reflects upon one single event, often where a mistake has been made or the outcome was not desired • Beneficial to encourage the reporting of errors or near-misses • <u>Must</u> adopt a no-blame policy • Example: never event in surgery (i.e. missed prophylactic antibiosis) or unexpected patient mortality

Figure 3.6 The four different types of clinical audit. Source: Adaptation from Mosedale 2019.

Identification of an Area for Improvement

For the audit to be valuable, the area selected for improvement needs to be one that is commonly encountered. Ultimately, the audit needs to be relevant to the practice, in addition to facilitating realistic and appropriate recommendations for implementations to enable improvement.

Selecting Criteria and Setting a Target

As part of the audit process, criteria must be decided upon. Often, these criteria are based upon best practice standards, informed by evidence produced from research. Alternatively, clinical discussions may help to identify desired practice standards. RCVS Knowledge (2021c) outlines a structure for deciding upon criteria using the acronym DREAM:

1. *Distinct:* Identify a specific area to focus your audit on. If your criteria are too broad, it will be difficult to create specific recommendations.
2. *Relevant:* Ensure that you consider an area that will be able to have a positive impact on the practice.
3. *Evidence-based:*[1] Literature searches to identify relevant literature to guide criteria formation are essential to inform evidence-based criteria.
4. *Achievable:* At this point, consideration should be given to what can be achieved bearing in mind the practice resources available.
5. *Measurable:* To be able to measure change, data gathered must be quantifiable.

The next step is to decide upon your target. This could be a specific number of cases or a period of time. If the practice sees a high number of cases, a time limit may be more appropriate. However, if cases are more limited, reaching an appropriate number should be identified and data collected until this is reached. Target setting should also be evidence-based, and a literature review should be conducted to help to inform your target. If the evidence-base is limited, a clinical discussion can be carried out to decide targets based upon caseload, experience, and nature of the improvements needing to be made. Alternatively, if the area has been audited before, the findings from this can act as a standard, and therefore can be used as a target for the next audit.

Data Collection

Data collection methods will depend on how you wish to conduct your audit. Data can be collected prospectively, meaning you gather data over a set period of time, or until you have reached the desired number, and can include patients, or events,

---

[1] NB: Some areas are not well researched. However, it is necessary to establish this by carrying out a broad search. If there are no published standards, you may use your own practice data (previous audits perhaps) as an evidence base for your criteria.

that match your criteria. Alternatively, data can be collected retrospectively, using information that has already been gathered, for example, within patient records.

Examples of how data can be collected prospectively include:

- client questionnaires/surveys
- staff questionnaires/surveys
- equipment performance records
- patient care forms, such as anaesthetic recovery sheets, CPR sheets, pain scale sheets and surgical safety checklists.

It may be valuable to brief all members of the team involved in data collection to ensure standardisation. This means that you are all looking for, and measuring, the same aspects of practice in the same way, ensuring that you gain an accurate clinical picture, and the recommendations are objective. Some tasks, such as pain assessment, may introduce subjectivity, however, this can be mediated using validated scales and an agreed criterion.

For each method, prospective and retrospective data is collected and then analysed as a data set.

Analyse Data

Once you have reached your target and have a wealth of data, you need to know what to do with it. Data analysis is the process of collating and interpreting the data you have collected. There are many different computer software programmes that can assist with this; Microsoft Excel is probably the most common. Presenting your data in charts or graphs will allow trends and patterns to be identified. At this point, you can compare your findings with the criteria and targets set prior to data collection.

Implement Change

In response to the data analysis, a team meeting should be held to discuss the findings. This will help to identify where changes need to be made. These will be individual to the practice; however, outcomes could include, but are not limited to, the creation of new documents such as checklists, SOPs, protocols, or alterations to current guidelines.

Re-audit

If it is decided that changes should be made and implemented, a second, follow-up audit should be carried out to measure their impact. This audit should utilise the same criteria and targets as the first, but data collection, analysis, and implementation of any changes should be undertaken. The impact should be positive, with the ultimate outcome being an improvement in the area of audit.

Review and Reflect

This stage is arguably the most important. The practice team should review the process of the audit to identify areas of strength and challenges faced. These should be discussed and considered for the next audit.

Barriers to Auditing

A large-scale review of 93 publications from the medical profession found that the five key barriers to auditing included lack of expertise, lack of resources, poor planning for the audit, and issues between team members and other organisational limitations; an additional barrier was identified as lack of time (Johnston et al. 2000). Within this audit, advantages of carrying out clinical audits were outlined: improved team communications, improved patient care, increased professional satisfaction, and improved administration. Similar results were found following a systematic review of published audits in the veterinary medical field, with perceived advantages including reduced clinical error, promotion of high standards of care, and teambuilding (Rose et al. 2016). Johnston et al. (2000) summarised disadvantages of auditing, which included diminished clinical ownership, fear of litigation, hierarchical suspicions, and professional isolation. Curtis (2020) concurs that barriers within veterinary medicine include those outlined by Johnston et al. (2000) as well as a lack of knowledge of RVNs as to the scientific process of data collection. RVNs should be reflecting upon and identifying these, for example knowledge gaps, and aim to develop skills to overcome them, an example of autonomous behaviour. Although the benefits of audit are evident, teams must ensure not to over-audit to reduce process lethargy in addition to overwhelming the practice(s) with data to analyse.

The RVN as a Political Leader

Many RVNs may not identify with the role of political leadership. However, as the role of the RVN evolves, and they take on greater responsibility within practice, demonstrating more autonomous behaviours and accepting accountability, it is imperative that they are champions of their own professional positions. Individual veterinary nurses should consider themselves as figureheads of change to drive high standards of care through the means we have already discussed throughout this chapter.

When thinking of politics, many will think of the Houses of Parliament, 10 Downing Street, and general elections. However, political leadership does not just mean campaigning with, or as, your local MP. For RVNs, it means being involved with regulatory body surveys and polls, and for some, involvement with RCVS VN Council or other organisations such as the BVNA, or being a part of professional working groups. These actions ultimately lead to RVNs being in positions to influence fundamental changes to many aspects of the governance of the veterinary nursing profession.

A fairly recent example of a political movement within veterinary nursing was the campaign to protect the title of Veterinary Nurse, as discussed previously within this chapter. Although this petition was not successful at the time, it clearly demonstrates that there is traction for change and for promotion of veterinary nursing. Involvement in professional politics is necessary by members of the veterinary workforce, specifically those enrolled on the Register, in order to advance the status of veterinary nurses.

There are many opportunities for veterinary nurses to be involved in politics associated with the profession. One example is to follow or become directly involved with the RCVS VN Council.

Replacing the Veterinary Nurses Committee in 2002, the RCVS VN Council assumes responsibility for veterinary nurse training, post-qualification awards, and registration of veterinary nurses. The Council is formed of elected and appointed RVNs, appointed veterinary surgeons, and lay persons. Key roles include:

- setting standards for training and education
- setting requirements for registration
- ensuring compliance with requirements of registration and conduct of veterinary nurses, including disciplinary proceedings
- recommending budgets and fees to the Finance and Resources Committee.

The RCVS is the regulatory body for RVNs, whilst the BVNA is the representative organisation. The BVNA also has an elected Council comprised only of RVNs and student veterinary nurses. Roles within BVNA Council are more flexible and are focused on individual members' interests and strengths but are united in raising awareness of the veterinary nursing role and advancing the profession.

VN Futures

VN Futures is an initiative that was set up by the RCVS and the BVNA in 2016, to map the future of the veterinary nursing profession. The RCVS Council and BVNA share goals of meeting the aims of the VN Futures initiative. Key objectives are centred around identification of challenges and barriers the profession may encounter and creating strategies to mitigate these. At the beginning, VN Futures set out to move through three phases, with phases one and two working to identify and refine key strategic issues. It is now on phase three, which is the delivery of the action plan. The VN Futures Ambitions are outlined in Figure 3.7.

Passion for advancement of the veterinary nursing profession is evident in abundance by virtue of numerous innovative initiatives, plans, and strategies which set out to promote awareness of the veterinary nursing role in addition to protection of the individuals working tirelessly each day to provide the highest standards of patient care.

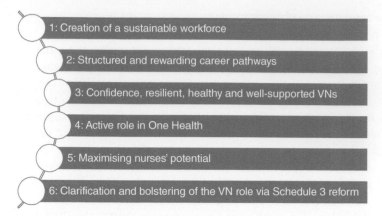

1: Creation of a sustainable workforce

2: Structured and rewarding career pathways

3: Confidence, resilient, healthy and well-supported VNs

4: Active role in One Health

5: Maximising nurses' potential

6: Clarification and bolstering of the VN role via Schedule 3 reform

Figure 3.7   VN Futures Ambitions. Source: Adapted from VN Futures 2016.

Changes and political movements will affect each and every RVN at some point, so remaining up to date with professional news is key to ensuring relevance and compliance with CPD requirements. Maintaining a political mindset and remaining open to change is important to facilitate advancement. Encouragement and support of colleagues to become active political members of various bodies can also foster a sense of achievement, professional ownership, and reward.

Ethics and the RVN

The development of veterinary nursing into a full profession has brought with it more engagement with ethical issues. Issues faced by veterinary nurses include breed specific health problems, convenience euthanasia, reporting malpractice and diversity in the profession. As veterinary nurses become more involved in policy-making and political issues, they must engage with the ethical challenges presented in this context. Veterinary nurses must not just consider 'what can I do' but 'what is the right thing for me to do'. In addition, the veterinary profession is coming to terms with the issues of compassion fatigue and moral injury. Compassion fatigue is the loss of empathy and compassion resulting from mental and physical exhaustion, whereas moral injury is the feeling of guilt and shame resulting from acting contrary to one's own moral compass. These feelings may be caused by the differences between what veterinary professionals feel is the right thing to do, and what they are required to do. These issues can lead to problems with mental health, struggles to manage at work, and people leaving the profession. In extreme cases, this may even lead to self-harm. Ethical decision-making can help ensure that nurses feel they have taken the best possible actions under the circumstances.

Philosophical Paradigms

Until recently ethics was rarely taught as a distinct or formal part of the veterinary nursing curriculum, so many nurses may be unfamiliar with ethical approaches and ways to apply them to the decision-making process. Here we summarise some key ethical theories that can be used to help evaluate ethical issues.

Deontology/duty-based ethics describes systems where some actions are right or wrong to perform, irrespective of the consequences. These may often be tied to religious beliefs. An example would be someone who believes euthanasia is morally wrong.

Utilitarianism/consequentialism are instead based on the idea that consequences are most important. When approaching a problem, one should look for a solution that creates the greatest happiness or welfare improvements for the largest number of people and/or animals.

Contractarianism is concerned with social contracts; that is, the duties we owe to other people due to the laws and social norms of our society. We can consider an issue based on what we believe we are obliged to do for the other parties, for example sharing all treatment options with a client regardless of our own preferences. A disadvantage of this approach is that it generally does not consider animals as stakeholders.

Virtue ethics approaches each issue with the question: What would a virtuous person do? Patience, honesty, and fairness are examples of virtues. In a given situation, the virtuous person would ask what the most honest or fair action is, depending on the virtues they espoused.

Rights-based ethics are similar to duty-based ethics in that there are certain rights that all humans have, which must be respected. Animal rights takes the position that there are no fundamental differences between humans and other sentient animals, and that therefore animals must have some rights as well. The challenge is in determining what these rights would be, and how to protect them. The declaration of animal sentience by the UK Government in 2021 is likely to change how sentience is defined in law, and may have long-term effects on the application of other animal legislation.

Each of these theories can be used as a lens to examine an ethical problem from a different approach. This can aid the veterinary nurse to develop a range of possible responses, and to help with understanding the motivations of other stakeholders. In many ways this approach is similar to that used when weighing up welfare concerns and trying to find a balance between conflicting necessities. They can also be used as a way to examine ethical decisions for consistency. For example, if you consider being fair to clients as an ethical priority, you can examine your policies and client care approach with this in mind and identify areas that may not be consistent with your principles. For example, your practice may offer discounts to clients in financial difficulty. Fairness would require you to develop a systematic approach to these situations so there was no bias in deciding who would and wouldn't be offered a discount. For example, how would clients prove they were experiencing financial difficulty, and how would the practice determine when to apply discounts?

Figure 3.8 shows how ethical thinking fits into the decision-making process. Firstly, it is necessary to identify all the stakeholders in any situation. This can include specific individuals (animals, clients, veterinary staff) or larger groups (businesses, organisations, the veterinary profession as a whole). For each

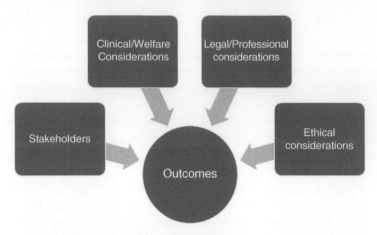

Figure 3.8   A framework for ethical decision-making.

stakeholder you need to determine what they would see as an acceptable solution to the issue. For example, a practice may prioritise client retention and prefer to avoid any solutions that might result in clients leaving the practice.

Secondly, any clinical and welfare concerns need to be addressed. This may be straightforward in clinical cases but can also involve broader aspects such as overall welfare of animals in a practice. When looking at issues such as breed specific health problems, this requires a degree of evaluation of the scope and severity of the issues to support the decision-making process.

Thirdly, legal, and professional aspects need to be considered. Veterinary nurses work within a legal framework and have their professional responsibilities set out in the RCVS Code of Professional Conduct for Veterinary Nurses. Any actions taken must not clash with these legal or professional requirements. There has been one publicly reported case where a registered veterinary nurse reported to a client that their animal had been euthanised as per their request, when actually the RVN had kept the animal. While this person may have considered that they were morally correct in this action, it was both illegal and unprofessional and they faced disciplinary action accordingly.

Many RVNs will be familiar with taking the above steps to resolve clinical and workplace issues. When the issues are less straightforward, or if there is conflict between one or more stakeholders, ethical analysis can take place. Using ethical theories, the possible outcomes suggested by the process can be analysed. RVNs can consider how to characterise their own viewpoint, and that of the other stakeholders. Is the issue that one party considers a certain action morally wrong, for example, euthanasia, whereas the other party sees it as the best overall welfare option? Perhaps the clash is over animal rights such as an animal's freedom to breed, versus the responsibility to minimise the number of unwanted pets in the world? Considering problems from these different viewpoints may not provide clear solutions, but it is helpful in determining how best to approach an issue with consideration for the values of each stakeholder, and in determining the approach most acceptable to all parties.

As the veterinary nursing profession develops, there is an increasing concern about the RVN's role within the wider veterinary profession. Veterinary nurses no longer simply concern themselves with issues within clinical practice; many veterinary nurses campaign passionately for animal welfare, for recognition of their profession, and to determine what role RVNs should play in the veterinary field as a whole. This framework (Figure 3.8) can also be applied to these larger questions. For example, a veterinary nurse might decide to start a campaign against online animal sales. They can consider the stakeholders (veterinary profession, welfare organisations, animals, sellers, owners), the welfare issues (animals going to unsuitable homes, etc.), and the legal issues (Animal Welfare Act 2006, Animal Welfare (Licensing of Activities Involving Animals) (England) Regulations 2018, etc.).

Ethical analysis at this point would help to determine the stated goals of the campaign and how it would frame its arguments. Ethical considerations are also important in issues of professional misconduct and whistleblowing, as discussed elsewhere in this chapter.

Summary

In summary, professional veterinary nursing is an extremely diverse, fascinating, and ever-evolving role. Each RVN should make an effort to understand themselves as a professional by seeking out and nurturing their professional identity in addition to understanding where that fits with the veterinary nursing and veterinary professions as overarching entities. Each RVN has the potential to initiate and monitor change to promote best practice and to lead their colleagues to discover new insights in patient care and well-being. It is essential that RVNs practise within their legal boundaries and thus they must have an astute awareness of them. They must consider the ethics of their practice in addition to the implications of their actions and be accountable for them. The role of the professional RVN is advancing; these are exciting times for veterinary nurses, with changes to what they are allowed to do on the horizon. It is important not to lose sight of where we have come from, and we must continue to adapt and learn to drive our profession forwards.

References

BVNA (2021a). Who we are. https://bvna.org.uk (accessed March 2021).

BVNA (2021b). Mission statement and values. https://bvna.org.uk/mission-statement-values (accessed April 2021).

Crowe, C. (2015). Recognising and dealing with bullying. *In Pract.* 37: 427–429.

Curtis, A. (2020). Clinical governance: quality improvement and clinical audits in practice. *The Veterinary Nurse* 11 (9): 388–399.

Curtis, E.A., de Vries, J., and Sheerin, F.K. (2011). Developing leadership in nursing: exploring core factors. *Br. J. Nurs.* 20 (5): 306–309.

Fraser, M. (2019). An overview of decision making in veterinary nursing. *Vet. Nurs.* 10 (9): 460–464.

Gov.uk (n.d.). Petition Parliament and the government. https://www.gov.uk/petition-government (accessed April 2021).

Johnston, G., Crombie, I.K., Alder, E.M. et al. (2000). Reviewing audit: barriers and facilitating factors for effective clinical audit. *BMJ Qual. Saf.* 9: 23–36.

Kerrigan, L. (2018). An introduction to veterinary nursing leadership part one: getting to know yourself. *Vet. Nurs.* 9 (9): 452–457.

Mason, T. and Whitehead, E. (2003). *Thinking Nursing.* Milton Keynes: Open University Press.

Mosedale, P. (2019). Clinical audit in veterinary practice – the role of the veterinary nurse. *Vet. Nurs.* 10 (1): 4–10.

RCVS (2014). Veterinary Nurse Conduct and Discipline Rules 2014. https://www.rcvs.org.uk/document-library/veterinary-nurse-conduct-and-discipline-rules-2014/ (accessed January 2022).

RCVS (2019). Continuing Professional Development Policy for Veterinary Nurses 2020. https://www.rcvs.org.uk/document-library/cpd-policy-for-vns/ (accessed January 2021).

RCVS (2020a). *Strategic Plan 2020–2024.* https://www.rcvs.org.uk/news-and-views/publications/rcvs-strategic-plan-2020-2024 (accessed April 2021).

RCVS (2020b). 20. Raising concerns about a colleague. https://www.rcvs.org.uk/setting-standards/advice-and-guidance/code-of-professional-conduct-for-veterinary-surgeons/supporting-guidance/whistle-blowing/#:~:text=20.7%20Certain%20whistle%2Dblowing%20is,employers%20if%20they%20whistle%2Dblow.&text=20.8%20Whistle%2Dblowing%20may%20be,the%20Act%20applies%20or%20not (accessed March 2021).

RCVS (2021a). RCVS Disciplinary Procedure. https://www.rcvs.org.uk/who-we-are/committees/veterinary-nurse-disciplinary-committee (accessed March 2021).

RCVS (2021b). What counts as CPD? https://www.rcvs.org.uk/faqs/what-counts-as-cpd-continued (accessed April 2021).

RCVS (2021c). Code of Professional Conduct for Veterinary Nurses. https://www.rcvs.org.uk/setting-standards/advice-and-guidance/code-of-professional-conduct-for-veterinary-nurses (accessed February 2021).

RCVS Knowledge (2021a). Veterinary nursing timeline. https://knowledge.rcvs.org.uk/heritage-and-history/history-of-the-veterinary-profession/veterinary-nursing-timeline (accessed March 2021).

RCVS Knowledge (2021b). QI, it's all part of the process. https://oncourse.rcvsk.org/courses/clinical-audit/modules/introduction-to-clinical-audit-3/lessons/qi-its-all-part-of-a-process-3 (accessed January 2021).

RCVS Knowledge (2021c). Setting a criteria to measure. https://oncourse.rcvsk.org/courses/clinical-audit/modules/performing-an-audit-3/lessons/setting-criteria-to-measure-4 (accessed February 2021).

Rose, N., Toews, L., and Pang, D.S.J. (2016). A systematic review of clinical audit in companion animal veterinary medicine. *BMC Vet. Res.* 12: 40. https://doi.org/10.1186/s12917-016-0661-4.

VN Futures (2016). VN Futures Report. www.vnfutures.org.uk (accessed April 2021).

Welsh, P. and Bayliss, S. (2013). Whistle-blowing explained: to be or not to be a whistle-blower, that is the question. *Vet. Nurs.* 3 (2): 122–126.

Further Reading

Pullen, S. and Gray, C. (2006). *Ethics, Law and the Veterinary Nurse.* Edinburgh: Elsevier Butterworth Heinemann.

Sandøe, P., Corr, S., and Palmer, C. (2015). *Companion Animal Ethics.* Oxford: Wiley Blackwell.

Useful Additional Resources

British Veterinary Nursing Association website: www.bvna.org.uk
Royal College of Veterinary Surgeons website: www.rcvs.org.uk/home
VN Futures website: www.vnfutures.org.uk

4 Clinical Advocacy – The RVN's Responsibility to the Patient and the Client

Kathy Kissick

What is Meant by the Term 'Advocacy'?

Advocacy is considered by many to be a relatively new and modern idea but the first consideration of patient advocacy was by Florence Nightingale, who talked about justice being amongst the most basic of human needs and one of the needs that could be provided by nurses. This was the beginning of the vital link between the patient and holistic nursing care.

All veterinary nurses want to deliver quality care to their patients, but this is not just knowing about diseases and their impact. The veterinary nurse can help clients to make informed decisions regarding the health of their pets and to assist them in navigating what may appear to the client to be complex veterinary health-care systems and decisions. They can help to translate medical terminology and guide them when they are having to make exceedingly difficult ethical decisions.

Advocacy is generally defined as defending the rights and properties of others, being the representative for the patient, defending their rights, protecting their interests, and contributing to decision-making regarding their care. Advocacy is often forgotten as a concept of veterinary nursing practice, one of those concepts that we all think we do daily with little consideration given to improvements that could be made. It is an ambiguous term when levelled at veterinary nursing as the generalised interpretation is used to describe the nurse–client relationship, but what about our patients? Where do they fit in?

What this Means for the Veterinary Nurse

Being a patient rights advocate is to be applauded but it encompasses so much more, it is about patient rights but also about nursing support to promote the patient's well-being, it is about communicating with your colleagues and your

Professionalism and Reflection in Veterinary Nursing, First Edition.
Edited by Sue Badger and Andrea Jeffery.
© 2022 John Wiley & Sons Ltd. Published 2022 by John Wiley & Sons Ltd.
Companion website: www.wiley.com/go/badger/professionalism-veterinary-nursing

clients about your patient, and it is an ethic of practice. Protecting our patients against unethical and illegal acts is only a small part of patient advocacy.

Clinical advocacy is seen by many as an ideal in nursing practice when indeed it should be a natural part of veterinary nursing. Veterinary nursing aspires to embrace autonomy of practice, it is a professional goal and if we, as a profession, are to work towards this goal then it is paramount that we enhance our patient care, making the veterinary nurse accountable for the veterinary nursing services accessible to our patients.

Any patient in our care is vulnerable and this is especially true for veterinary patients as there is no one to speak on their behalf so the nurse must be prepared to become the voice of the defenceless.

Our patients cannot participate in the decision-making process by speaking up and advocating for themselves, they do not have the ability to do so. For this reason, interpersonal skills and relationships with the client, which involve a professional rapport, are so important.

Enforcing patient advocacy means that the veterinary nursing profession can be viewed as critical in the improvement of the quality of patient care, and in addition, this role will help to enrich the veterinary nursing profession.

Veterinary nurses who successfully advocate for their clients and patients also promote the healing process, which is facilitated by taking responsibility, empowerment, communication, honesty, integrity, and adopting a moral stance.

RVN's enter the profession because they have a desire to help others, and this must include the client and their pet(s). Preventing and managing suffering is a significant part of what they do daily, and this can be achieved at the physical, emotional, and psychological level. Veterinary nurses should be prepared to support their patients, clients and, sometimes, their extended families, as advocates for their well-being.

Acting as an advocate for our patients is a delicate, fine line to walk, which can be problematic and challenging for the novice, unassertive veterinary nurse. Acting in an adversarial or in an oppositional role for the rights of your patients may lead to animosity within the veterinary healthcare team, especially if you are questioning the hierarchical systems, your employers, or the veterinary surgeon in charge of the clinical case. Advocacy should never be considered as being concerned with conflict for its own sake, it should be a positive constructional activity that is an essential part of the veterinary nurse's role. The veterinary nurse should always have the patient's best interests at heart. Patients must be made a priority and RVN's must stand up for the rights of their patients and defend their needs and in doing so they must be prepared to put personal feelings or preferences aside.

Patient Advocacy

So how do we work towards this personal relationship with our patients and the holistic veterinary nursing approach to patient care? Veterinary nurses see their patients in totality, the complete patient. In this respect we mimic what Florence

Nightingale did; she considered advocacy to be the art of making sure the patient was in the best condition but always ensured that it was the best condition for that individual patient, which is an enabler to determining the nursing actions and care required.

Patient advocacy is much more complicated in veterinary nursing than human-centred nursing because of the need to triangulate the communication and informed decision-making with the client but maintaining the patient in the pivotal role. The veterinary nurse is promoting, advocating for, and protecting the rights and health and safety of the patient in their care, but must seek the owner's consent and work under the auspices of the attending veterinary surgeon.

If you cannot see the world through the eyes of your clients and your patients, how can you know what they need? Asking the right questions and probing to understand the answers from your client is the first step towards finding out what your patient's specific needs are.

Veterinary nursing is a profession, but many RVN's feel emasculated because of the need to work 'under veterinary direction', as stated in The Veterinary Surgeons Act 1966 (Schedule 3 Amendment) Order 2002, but for a positive culture of ownership there are many essential characteristics that the profession must adopt if its members want to change. The RVN needs, as an individual professional, to embrace a degree of emotional positivity and self-empowerment as well as being fully engaged with both the profession and its stakeholders, to enable a culture of ownership and positive change.

To be a successful advocate for your patients you must demonstrate compassion and your workplace needs to give you permission to act on this as patient-centred practice should always come first, permission to spend extra time with a recovering patient should be the norm not the exception.

The ability to maintain patience and gain your patient's trust is an essential skill and all the veterinary healthcare encounters that our patients undergo should allow us to build on that trust by ensuring that all experiences are as painless and non-confrontational as possible.

Paying close attention to your patients with thorough assessments combined with the ability to identify ways to maintain patient comfort ensures that the veterinary nurse will succeed in picking up subtle but vital signs that something is wrong and be able to catch them early enough.

Sally Gadow, a human nurse, devised a model of existential advocacy and this stated that the process of advocating involves multidimensional actions (Gadow 1980) This cannot be achieved in veterinary practice unless the veterinary nurse works in an empowering veterinary environment that views advocacy as the ideal for a successful nurse to patient and nurse to client relationship.

Advocacy underpins the veterinary nurse's decision-making experience and can be considered as a means for individuals to be empowered to express their opinions. By defending the patients' rights veterinary nurses are upholding animal welfare, as their role of advocate empowers the client and the patient, who are otherwise unable to assert their own needs. The veterinary nurse generally uses a value decision model where they help the patient with their needs, interests, and choices through the client. They are making informed critical organisational decisions that are also appropriate to meeting the needs of the patient. Value-based decision-making enables the veterinary nurse to identify the most critical decisions that they are facing, what information is required to make those decisions and the best time to make them.

Veterinary nurses must be strong patient advocates and use their own experienced professional voices to determine individual patient needs and the best interests of the patients in their care and promote those interests using their own voices. They should notice small changes in their patients, as these may be first indications that problems are arising or that there are limited responses to the treatment being administered. It is important that these changes are shared with the team, it is your duty to speak out in a timely manner, especially if your patient's safety is at risk. We are in a unique position where, as veterinary nurses, we are responsible for most of our patients care and more importantly the quality of that care.

Minute by minute care should be discussed with the veterinary surgeon in charge of the case and this is especially important when considering pain relief. It is for us to make nursing care recommendations on the nursing management of our cases and it is at these times that it is important that we use critical thinking and observations as well as the skills of interpretation, communication, and reflection to act as the patient advocate. Our interactions with our patients will determine adjustments to treatments and pain management, nursing, or feeding regimes, changes to drug protocols or the addition of other drugs to the treatment protocol.

As a veterinary nurse, you are responsible for continuous monitoring of the patients in your care but in the UK at present RVN's do not have the freedom to prescribe, diagnose, or initiate treatments though we do have the freedom and responsibility to administer agreed treatment changes and alterations to treatments and analgesia.

When veterinary nurses have a voice then thoughts and skills are valued, leading to a positive team environment. This in turn means that patients receive better care, and the veterinary nurse is satisfied that they are doing everything that they can. RVN's are, of course, ethically obliged to speak up and ask questions when problems arise.

Client Advocacy

Many clients are anxious and confused when their pet is ill, and a calm veterinary nurse can help them to steer their way through the system and assist them with clinical communications with the veterinary surgeon. Nurses educate the clients about their pet's diagnostic tests and procedures whilst always being aware of how culture and ethnicity can impact on the experience of the client and their pet. Veterinary nurses can integrate all aspects of patient care, address all concerns, uphold standards, and ensure that positive outcomes remain the ultimate goal.

Advocacy also means having respect for the other person's views as fellow human beings. The client and the patient deserve to have their dignity, privacy, and choices protected and this is most evident when dealing with end-of-life cases; the veterinary nurse must not impose their values onto the client or patient and by doing so influence their decisions adversely.

Conflict occurs sometimes between the interests of the patient and the interests of the client who is paying for the treatment. Working in a multidisciplinary role as a veterinary nurse we cannot assume a passive role and need to employ good communication skills. Advocacy may place you out of your comfort zone at times and a veterinary nurse may have to command a degree of courage to speak out, but we must remember that we are dealing with sentient beings in our care.

Advocacy Within the Team Context

How your clients perceive the quality of their experience will be determined by your care and compassion towards their pet and this needs to spill over into a unified veterinary care team that puts the patient first.

Every member of the team must demonstrate a degree of assertiveness particularly when they recognise that a patient needs help or is in trouble and even more so if they have suggestions for a solution. The veterinary nurse must nurture a culture of listening and remember that every member of the veterinary team is valuable and has something helpful to offer to every case, everyone has a voice and should be listened to.

Veterinary nursing leadership is important for every patient as someone must take charge of nursing care and maintain an overview of the patients going into consultations, into theatre, into recovery or discharged for home care. A lack of nursing leadership will give rise to many nursing personnel working independently to achieve their own goal. Veterinary nurses must train themselves to think ahead, to embrace teamwork, to have situational awareness where they can maintain an understanding of what is going on around them at every moment and use that information to mitigate risk and build decision-making into all aspects of their patient care.

The potential for error should not be ringfenced to poor performance or weakness, as you cannot eliminate human error in totality from veterinary nursing practice, but through accountability and appropriate training as well as implementation of systems, and processes. This approach serves to identify minor errors, which can be fixed before they become harmful or critical errors.

If nurses are aware of things that have gone wrong or are going wrong, can they voice it in your practice? Can they speak up or do they see it as not their place to do so?

Visit the companion website where you will find additional resources for this chapter (www.wiley.com/go/badger/professionalism-veterinary-nursing) and carry out Exercise 4.1.

Situational awareness gives us, as the patient advocate, the ability to anticipate patient needs by knowing what is happening, why it is happening and what is likely to happen next, it gives us the 'big picture'.

Non-technical skills training on decision-making, situational awareness and teamwork helps us to understand our behaviour better and to anticipate how we may react and behave in crucial and critical moments. We are more likely to stop and think in emergency situations and to speak up if we have been trained and encouraged to do so.

Many RVN's are present from the first contact with patients, especially if they are community nurses or run their own clinics, and they are responsible for establishing regular, continued, and integrated nursing care. The responsibility of the veterinary nurse is not just limited to that of advocate for the vulnerable patient, they also need to provide patient-focused care and contribute to bringing better value to the ever-increasing costs of veterinary care. A veterinary nurse should be able to perceive what is happening to their patient, understand the situation, and plan for the possible implications. If distracted the veterinary nurse will tend to miss cues of deterioration and any signs of the patient's status becoming critical, leading to the need for additional examinations and an altered nursing care plan.

Patient or nursing advocacy, at its pinnacle, is an advanced nursing care procedure that exemplifies the professional power of nursing and is dominant in providing safe and effective nursing care, but nursing advocacy can be considered a two-pronged methodology that should be approached and considered by the whole nursing team:

a. patient empathy where the nurse is understanding and sympathetic to the needs of that patient and feels close to the patient
b. protecting the patient; this is critical in veterinary nursing where it must include patient care, prioritising patient health and completion of the care process.

It may be over-simplistic to give a single definition for patient advocacy, but we need to be mindful that protecting the patient is a key factor in patient advocacy. Veterinary nurses are responsible for protecting patients against inadequate veterinary healthcare provided by other team members. The support systems must be in place in all veterinary settings, to ensure that clinical advocacy is viewed as an inclusive and supported role that can be undertaken by all team members.

Veterinary nurses sometimes find it difficult to challenge veterinary surgeons or senior members of the team for fear of confrontation, hostility, or due to their personal lack of confidence or resilience; it is not usually expected that 'just a veterinary nurse' will question or confront a veterinary surgeon. There is often a strict occupational hierarchy where generally the veterinary nurse is subordinate to the veterinary surgeon, and this hierarchical structure is a severe obstruction to raising concerns on medical decisions and is detrimental to patient care. 'Just' a veterinary nurse is such a destructive phrase; when the word 'just' is used in this descriptive context, it is a most unjust word, which strips us as a profession of our dignity and our professional status.

> Visit the companion website where you will find additional resources for this chapter (www. wiley.com/go/badger/professionalism-veterinary-nursing) and carry out Exercise 4.2.

Advocacy and Accountability

Veterinary nurses are held accountable by the RCVS Code of Professional Conduct for Veterinary Nurses and do have restrictions imposed upon them by The Veterinary Surgeons Act 1966 (Schedule 3 Amendment) Order 2002. A Code of Conduct is a framework for behaviour and as such is an outline of how the profession considers its veterinary nurses should behave towards patients, clients, each other, and society. However, many of the perceived cultural problems can be overcome if the veterinary nurse takes up the challenge of accountability, which in turn will enhance their role as a patient advocate and empower them as a professional.

The veterinary world of today is technologically challenging, complex, and dynamic and the veterinary nurse must look beyond their job description, take personal ownership for the values and mission of their practice or organisation, and nurture the role in order to hold themselves accountable in all aspects of their work.

Being accountable is not just following your job description; you also must be accountable for your attitudes at work and the way you treat your clients, patients, and others encountering you. Accountability means accepting responsibility for the actions you take to provide the correct care for your patients. The RCVS professional declaration, taken at the point of RVN registration, outlines the rights and responsibilities of the veterinary nurse and, as previously mentioned, the RCVS Code of Professional Conduct for Veterinary Nurses sets out professional veterinary nurses' responsibilities to ensure the health and welfare of animals committed to their care.

Living the values of veterinary nursing through our Code of Conduct is a powerful tool that will enhance the importance of being patient-centred in everything we do. Our Code of Conduct provides a clear structure but, just as important, it emphasises the need to do the right thing for our patients, for the right reasons.

> Visit the companion website where you will find additional resources for this chapter (www. wiley.com/go/badger/professionalism-veterinary-nursing) and carry out Exercise 4.3.

Sharing a common set of professional values facilitates a degree of individual flexibility whilst also enabling the individual practitioner to use these core values as well as their personal values to inform their interactions with colleagues, patients, and clients.

In addition to the Code of Conduct, personal values will influence how a veterinary nurse treats others including the patients in their care. Core values define who you are and what you stand for and interlinked with these is integrity – in other words, doing the right thing even when no one is watching. Professional integrity is absent if, for example, clients, or colleagues overhear gossiping or complaining, and if this becomes institutional within a professional environment it leads to a situation where core values are undermined.

Our patients always deserve the absolute best of care and for this to happen veterinary nurses need to adopt a sense of ownership of their patient's care, ownership of their role, and ownership of their profession. Negativity cannot be switched on and off at choice without it creeping into everyday working life in the practice and it is this negative atmosphere that our clients sense rather than the cloak of empathy, care, and compassion that we should be generating. Accountability on its own will not produce an engaged and committed veterinary nurse who has their patients' needs as a priority and who wishes to nurture a culture of ownership.

Accountability means accepting responsibility for the actions that you take to provide care for your patients, and you must not forget to include your clients in that empowerment.

- Moral accountability cannot be demanded or measured, and it is the art of being accountable to oneself.
- Ethical accountability is being accountable to those we live or work with.
- Professional accountability must underpin your relationship with patients, clients, and the profession.

As a veterinary nurse these three genres of accountability need to be observed and understood at all levels of our work.

Accountability and responsibility are intricately connected but do not always go together; you can decide upon an action in a given set of circumstances and accountability means that the action or decision can be professionally defended. To be professionally accountable as an advocate for your patients you must take personal and professional responsibility.

Veterinary nurses must acknowledge their limits of professional competence and only undertake and accept responsibility for those activities in which they are competent, although there will be occasions when transferrable skills can be drawn upon, for example small animal skills transferrable to equine in a first aid situation or nursing skills that are extended into the role of the community nurse.

The UK regulatory body, the RCVS, guides the RVN in their day-to-day work, but each individual nurse must be the judge of any circumstances where this guidance might apply, and this is especially pertinent when work is delegated and as such accountability is clearly recognised. When supervising student veterinary nurses and colleagues you must make clear judgements about their level of skills and competence to ensure that they cause no harm to the patients or others, whilst those students accepting delegated work, must decide when they can accept responsibility. It must be remembered that ignorance is no defence, and neither is just following orders. A supportive work place environment will allow all members of the nursing team to accept responsibility for the actions they take to provide veterinary nursing care.

You are personally accountable for your actions and your omissions when working as a veterinary nurse and you must be able to justify your decisions even if given instructions by another person. It is imperative, then, that you consider the actions you take when nursing your patients, especially if a task or procedure is delegated to you. Being blamed and being accountable are not the same thing, and if this is the perception of staff members in a working environment it may mean that the individuals in question are over-defensive, through lack of confidence, or that a blame culture exists. This will result in individual veterinary nurses and the profession as a whole, becoming over reliant on protocols; it does not generate the ethos of critical thinking, reflection, and clinical judgement.

Accountability is intrinsic in our day-to-day work and allows a veterinary nurse to take pride in the transparency of veterinary nursing practice. Justifying your actions to others and recording and documenting all nursing care and its delivery, including omissions and the reasons for these, plus the outcomes of this care, means that you are realising your accountability.

Caring for your patients in an empathetic, sensitive, and compassionate manner whilst being aware of the relationship between the patient and the client, as well as recognising the client-bond and demonstrating a strong respect for the client, is a good example of ethical accountability.

Sometimes we must make quick decisions so that our patient will not suffer and we rely on intuition rather than guidelines, and in accounting for our actions we realise the enormity of the situation and the possible consequences. It is on these occasions that the development from novice to experienced nurse is most apparent, as the latter will have acted with professional, legal, and ethical accountability.

The Need for Empowerment to Support Advocacy

The use of a reflective approach to learning is a powerful tool for the veterinary nurse, who is engaging with new experiences throughout their career, but with new experiences, mistakes may be made. We learn from others, but to build confidence and resilience in the veterinary nursing team there needs to be a 'no blame' culture within the veterinary practice community and an ethos of wanting everyone to do well and develop both professionally and personally.

Empowerment is not something that is just given, it is a choice that must be made, and with it comes a degree of autonomy and self-determination. Once you have grasped empowerment you will have the ability to effectively motivate yourself and others to accomplish positive outcomes in veterinary nursing practice.

Once the veterinary nurse is elevated to a leadership position they can demonstrate this when making professional judgements in day-to-day nursing activities. Empowerment is quite different, though: it is a purposeful stimulus that is shared with others in the team, it incorporates the ability to motivate and organise oneself and others to realise positive outcomes, both in nursing practice and in the veterinary work environment. Empowerment of a veterinary nursing team will influence staff morale, patient care quality, patient safety, and ultimately staff retention. Veterinary nurses should enhance their leadership skills and become positive change makers, upgrade their knowledge through appropriate continued professional development, and embrace evidence-based veterinary nursing. Strive to make veterinary nursing an empowered profession and high-quality care and being a patient advocate will fall into place.

Empowerment synergises with patient advocacy, with many of the qualities overlapping:

- decision-making – we are making nursing decisions for every patient in our care
- autonomy – the veterinary nurse is a semi-autonomous nursing practitioner
- manageable workload – we all want to spend that extra time advocating and caring for our patients and their owners
- fairness – the veterinary nurse must treat everyone, including their patients and owners with fairness and integrity
- reward and recognition – veterinary nurses who are recognised for their work and feel appreciated will work better and the quality of care given to their patients will be the gold standard.

The veterinary nurse in the twenty-first century is required to have enormous amounts of energy and diligence. Regardless of the environment that they work in or the work challenges that envelop them, they must demonstrate flexibility in adapting to change in work and in professional relationships. Veterinary nurse leaders must be role models who do not sidestep problems but exhibit moral courage and commitment to their patients whilst directly addressing any challenges.

Autonomy in Veterinary Nursing

A semi-autonomous profession is one that requires a degree of advanced knowledge and skills. As UK veterinary nurses we have a minimal degree of control over some elements of our work. The RCVS carries out its functions under an Act of Parliament and makes rules, regulations, and byelaws. The original Royal Charter of 1844 was superseded by the Supplemental Charter of 1967, and this was then replaced by a new supplemental Charter in 2015.

The Royal Charter 2015 was formally granted and issued by the Queen and received the great Seal of the Realm. This fulfilled one of the profession's long-term goals of having a robust regulatory system in place for UK veterinary nurses. In doing so it recognised them as genuine, committed professionals, dedicated to proper conduct and professional development.

From the point of student registration, veterinary nurses are semi-autonomous and accountable practitioners. This role develops as the veterinary nurse progresses from student to qualified nurse and the changes along the way may be fraught, particularly if the professional responsibilities increase but the extent of these accountabilities leads to anxiety alongside the excitement of an advancing career.

As a semi-autonomous professional, the veterinary nurse should be allowed to act based on their knowledge and experience. If you leave a veterinary nurse powerless then they will become ineffective, their nursing role will become strained, and the result will be occupational burnout.

Teamwork and autonomy, including semi-autonomy, are intertwined and this close interaction of veterinary teamwork and autonomy leads to a nursing synergy.

Autonomy in nursing is the authority to use professional knowledge and judgement to make a decision and take actions that are consistent with the professional standards. To undertake this the veterinary nursing profession needs to develop greater self-direction, self-determination, and independence. To develop from the semi-autonomous professional role, the veterinary nurse needs to cultivate the holistic view and be confident enough to demonstrate their levels of knowledge and of patient care and hence are more than capable of making a nursing judgement or decision.

Professional autonomy is defined as a professional having the power over the practice of their discipline, and although veterinary nursing is not yet in this position in totality, veterinary nurses can take control of their ability to act according to their knowledge and judgement. They need to take control over the nursing context and be prepared to influence decision-making about their clinical practice by supporting it with evidence-based veterinary nursing research. This will inevitably result in improved veterinary nurse satisfaction and improved patient outcomes.

Clinical autonomy, that is, the authority, freedom, and discretion to make judgements about patient care, should be the objective of the veterinary nursing profession. We are already able to demonstrate control over our clinical practice with the authority, freedom, and discretion granted to us to make decisions in the context of organisational structure, policies, and procedures within our professional environment.

Veterinary nurses need to draw upon their knowledge and experience as they advance from novice to expert, a process that requires engaging with ever more challenging tasks. As previously discussed, they must do this with personal insight and knowledge of what they are capable of undertaking.

Veterinary nurses make autonomous decisions regarding their patients every day. Examples include:

- turning their patients to prevent hypostatic pneumonia
- taking blood and running haematology tests
- delegating help from the team to assist with lifting and walking non-ambulatory patients.

The level of autonomy conferred upon the RVN is influenced not only by the RCVS Code of Professional Conduct for Veterinary Nurses and the Veterinary Surgeons Act 1966 but also by the relationship with the veterinary surgeon or veterinary provider. There is most definitely a negative impact on the patient and the veterinary nursing team if the veterinary nurse is completely reliant on the veterinary surgeon to give instructions on all the intricacies of nursing care.

The veterinary nurse needs to be assertive and advocate for their patients, and offer the veterinary team ideas, relevant evidence-based veterinary nursing techniques, and best practices.

Wider Effects of Advocacy Within the Clinical Environment

When a veterinary nurse is working in a veterinary healthcare environment where they can make independent nursing care decisions based on their patients' needs everyone benefits; the team, the client, and the patient, who receives the best quality, safe nursing care. Veterinary nurses must advocate for safe, competent, and ethical care of their patients and the veterinary care team must work together in the best interests of the patients. Questioning and reflecting on the care of patients should never be a point-scoring or undermining exercise but should be undertaken with a strong team cohesion to promote patient well-being and enhance recovery. Working within a supportive interdisciplinary team, no matter what size the veterinary practice is, will increase the confidence of individual nursing staff and this positive exposure will promote high-quality patient care. Collaborative working is important in veterinary nursing in order to ensure adequate and suitable delivery of veterinary nursing services, which will also promote exemplary patient care. It is often challenging to interact with colleagues and veterinary care professionals in clinical settings, and being hesitant to speak out is often an element of the early stages of professional development.

Developing the qualities of non-challenging assertiveness and confidence in your abilities are factors that will support you when speaking out on behalf of your patients. Being a confident nurse who will speak up on behalf of patients in your care leads to improved patient care and positive experiences in the work environment.

Lacking confidence and underdeveloped assertiveness makes it difficult to advocate for patients, and this is frustrating when you are aware that you could have an impact on their care. Many veterinary nurses are unsure about the concept of advocacy and how to put it into practice in the day-to-day rigours of veterinary practice.

We all need to be prepared to push at the boundaries of our comfort zones in order to continue to grow in confidence and develop new strategies to improve the delivery of care by means of good time management and continuously reviewing common medications and conditions relevant to the cases that we are nursing. The application of an ethos of continuous professional development will lead to increased knowledge, and acquisition and repetition of new skills leads to improved confidence.

It is hard to be confident and advocate for a patient in your care if you are unable to communicate effectively with the client and your colleagues in order to identify needs and relay them to others within the veterinary care team. Veterinary nurses, in professional settings or in other organisations, exercise power in making professional judgements in all their day-to-day activities but face many barriers when they cannot always understand what their patients need because they are often poor communicators. In these cases, they must monitor and communicate the needs that are observable, and this normally starts with the patient's ability to feed and groom themselves and the need for pain relief. This starting point can be improved upon by collaborating with clients as this ensures that the veterinary nurse is also empowering them to be involved in their pet's care.

The complexity of veterinary healthcare has grown enormously with biomedical advances, an ageing pet population, regulatory activities, and client expectations as well as increased veterinary nursing responsibilities, and this has often equated to the boundaries between professions becoming blurred.

Interprofessional conflict and tensions between veterinary surgeons and veterinary nurses generates inconsistencies, especially when related to boundaries of authority and jurisdiction. Veterinary nurses need support to progress with new innovative patient care and work decisions. They should be encouraged and given the freedom to make important patient care and nursing decisions. They should not be placed in a position of having to do things that conflict with their nursing judgement. Developing confidence in selected nursing roles is vital for strong advocacy, and effective communication with clients, colleagues and stakeholders will naturally follow.

Employing veterinary nursing practitioners with a higher or advanced level of RVN qualification, who are engaged to complement veterinary surgeons in a close interprofessional team, could be a plausible strategic move within the professions to expand the professional role of the veterinary nurse and could be implemented without compromising the quality of veterinary pet care or patient outcomes. Extending the role of the veterinary nurse will challenge the professional identity of both veterinary nurses and veterinary surgeons and some people may struggle to maintain traditional professional boundaries, but controlled task delegation by the veterinary surgeon to the veterinary nurse practitioner leaves the veterinary surgeon free to manage more complex cases.

The true nature of nursing involves the critical thinking required to understand what is happening to the patient both physiologically and mentally, why various tasks are being performed, and the anticipatory versus the actual outcomes for that patient. It is not just about the veterinary nurse noticing changes in symptoms but also understanding that these may be indications of deeper problems. Catching these changes early and knowing what to expect is a skill that comes with experience but it should be an objective for professionals at all levels, not least because of its importance in maximising good patient care.

Communicating concerns to the rest of the veterinary team does not mean that you are making a diagnosis but are using the patient data and observations made about that patient to make nursing care decisions and care plan changes on a continual basis. When speaking to a veterinary surgeon about a concern, the veterinary surgeon should anticipate that you will give a recommendation on how to proceed with nursing care. Once it leaves the practice, a plan of care for the patient is essential; clients need to be empowered to handle the complex care regimes that may be required in some medical and surgical cases. Owners need to know how to care for their pets once they return home as well as how to look for the subtle changes that indicate improvement or deterioration of the pet's condition. In addition, veterinary nurses should be prepared to teach clients in other contexts, for example on flea or worm treatment, and to use their knowledge and experience to inform the general public.

The RVN needs to be prepared to take on the mantle of educator as there is much to teach the owners of sick patients as well as prophylactic care to clients in general, plus an enormous need to educate the public.

The veterinary nurse should always aim to provide holistic care, so be prepared to treat the whole patient and the client family including any extended family members. Time constraints are often a barrier, but pet health care can extend to far beyond the signs and symptoms that brought the client into the clinic in the first place. Community and district nursing allows a veterinary nurse to nurture in a much broader context and it enables the client to be confident in the care given as well as to be assisted with the emotional support required when a pet is sick.

Many fundamental tasks are undertaken by the veterinary nurse and specific procedures and protocols need focused attention; we must make sure that we do no harm to our patients when undertaking veterinary nursing procedures. Assessment of patients and consequential actions must be well thought out to balance the clinical requirements that need to be performed with precision alongside the emotional effort involved in being an RVN. To be an outstanding veterinary nurse the initial assessment process that leads to nursing activities and procedures must be well considered and competently accomplished.

All practising veterinary nurses have a responsibility to learn about technology trends, new veterinary nursing procedures, and veterinary science advancements. We must use assessment skills to uncover underlying issues, how they impact our patients, and the nursing care required to alleviate pain and suffering. To consider the countless variables, the possible treatments, the interventional choices, anticipating the worst and responding decisively when needed is key to being your patient's advocate. Veterinary nursing is a diverse profession where you must be prepared to put your own distinctive talents and your experiences to good use.

The Delivery of Nursing Care Within the Community

Home care planning is essential to determine the specific skilled nursing or client care a patient may need once discharged. It should consider every element of the patient's needs and the home environment to determine the best course of care. Patient welfare is considered by looking at the numerous components that make up the individual patient environment and routine.

- Consider the patient's background and what event or events led to this patient needing home care. This may include an event that has also impacted greatly on the owner.
- Identify the factors that will help build an understanding of how the veterinary nurse will need to interact and communicate with the patient and the family.

- Observe and reflect on the patient's activities of daily life and consider if help will be needed in standing, walking, getting into the car or up the steps, for example.
- Revisit existing or past medical conditions including those affecting sight or hearing as well as chronic and acute conditions.
- Deliberate over behavioural conditions, aggression, or separation anxiety, and remember to understand that these will influence the requirements needed to optimise the patient's living environment and ultimately optimise the road to recovery.
- Consider exercise, rehabilitation, and an exercise regime along with additional therapeutic equipment that may improve the quality of care.

Community home care veterinary nurses must provide care to patients under the guidance of a veterinary surgeon. Performing regular visits to monitor the patient's condition, assess wounds, change dressings, and assess improvements must all be reported and communicated back to the veterinary surgeon in charge of the case after each visit.

Multidimensional veterinary nursing home health care integrates research, education, proper use of resources, and the quality of care provided with team collaboration and ethical principles. It is a unique field of veterinary nursing and is the pinnacle of autonomous nursing and clinical advocacy.

Florence Nightingale was an early pioneer in evidence-based and research nursing and she relentlessly pursued greater knowledge to initiate and influence change. We are the guardians of our veterinary nursing profession and must use veterinary nursing research to drive change in the profession. The veterinary nurse practitioner would be an advanced and experienced veterinary nurse trained to assess patient needs, undertake and interpret diagnostic and laboratory tests, make a nursing diagnosis, and formulate and prescribe treatment plans. The veterinary nurse practitioner would focus on disease prevention and health education as well as placing a unique emphasis on the health and well-being of the whole patient.

Veterinary nurses are highly effective at managing chronic diseases and their care is well structured and of the highest quality. This could be further expanded to a more focused approach to areas such as coronary care, community care, patient screening, and the provision of suitable health promotion advice. The extension of the role of the veterinary nurse within the veterinary healthcare team would lead to many questions regarding legal liability if the care of a patient were to be fully discharged from the veterinary surgeon to the veterinary nurse. The dynamics influencing the extension of the veterinary nurse role are extremely complex, but the following aspects of progressive veterinary nursing must be considered:

- new technology, the portability of medical and veterinary web-based hardware for learning the advancement of bio- and pharmaco-therapeutics to replace invasive mechanical procedures, for example, chemotherapy replacing surgical intervention and excision
- veterinary healthcare information with web-based infrastructures facilitating access and providing support for the practising veterinary nurse

- complementary therapies that can be seamlessly integrated into existing clinical options to bring clinical value to the veterinary nursing care provided to patients
- the modern veterinary nurse needs to exhibit flexible skill sets that will enhance the care of individual cases.

The expansion of nurse prescribing in human nursing has been reported to have benefited patients, improved public health, and aided health care professionals in many ways. The opportunity to incorporate prescribing into the nursing role would seem an obvious progression for the experienced veterinary nurse; however, a number of hurdles to this increase in responsibility can be identified. These may be partly due to institutional, organisational, and resource factors as well as personal and professional attitudes. However, if some of the obstacles could be removed, if best practice could be readily implemented, and if communication and support networks could be further facilitated between the veterinary surgeon, the client, and the veterinary nurse, then the veterinary nurse prescriber role could begin to evolve.

Veterinary nurse prescribing incidents or potential issues that could affect patient safety appear to be the biggest concerns. However, the need for effective education, supervision, and auditing of veterinary nurse prescribing work and the initial imposition of limitations on the authorisation to prescribe would alleviate many of these risks. As nurse prescribers, there is a heightened risk of veterinary nurses becoming 'overly medicalised', so it is important that they must continue to retain traditional nursing roles in any future prescribing developments.

Perhaps the initial step into the world of prescribing would be for the veterinary nurse to become a supplementary prescriber where they are able to prescribe, in partnership with their veterinary surgeon, any medicine, including a limited range of controlled drugs. Veterinary nurse prescribers would rely to a greater or lesser extent on team working and the act of nurse prescribing would enhance teamwork between the nurses and the veterinary surgeons.

Many of the perceived challenges of retaining veterinary nurses in practice and providing a career pathway with empowerment and clinical autonomy would start to disappear with the introduction of the concept of veterinary nurse prescribers. Furthermore, there would be benefits, in relation to their personal development and feelings of personal reward, satisfaction at being able to provide total patient care, benefits related to freedom in decision-making, and enhancements in responsibility and autonomy. The ability to see their patients' care from beginning to end would be valued in the context of seamless continued care and more efficient use of time.

Conclusion

Empowerment, within the law and our Code of Conduct, allows the veterinary nurse to do the right thing for their patients and each other; so, do not sit around waiting, do what Florence Nightingale advocated and ensure that your workplace is an empowered place where veterinary nurses are doing the right thing for their patients because they have the knowledge, the courage, and the perseverance to do so.

Reference

Gadow, S. (1980). *Existential Advocacy: Philosophical Foundations of Nursing*. Washington, DC: NLN Publications.

5 The Veterinary Nurse's Role in Supporting the Client

Jill Macdonald

Introduction

Veterinary nurses hold a key role in the vet-led team; within practice, in provision of supportive healthcare to animals, in educating and supporting animal owners and future veterinary nurses, and in society. Their role is constantly evolving and developing, and veterinary nurses desire, and are being granted, a higher level of responsibility, accountability, and recognition for the work they perform.

This chapter will explore the differing ways in which veterinary nurses support clients, through effective and empathic communication, reinforcing client advocacy, offering veterinary healthcare advice and guidance, and helping clients through the difficult process of palliative and end-of-life care.

The chapter is written from the perspective of clinical small animal nursing as the default, but much of the content is generic and can be applied to all contexts of veterinary nursing.

One Health

There is no one, internationally agreed definition of One Health, although several suggested definitions can be sourced (Mackenzie and Jeggo 2019); however, the ideals of One Health embrace the concept of a holistic, transdisciplinary, multisectoral approach to healthcare, including consideration of the human, animal, and environmental factors.

Animals, animal companionship, and additional factors such as dog ownership assisting in health and fitness, can help us to see why the veterinary team has significant value in the One Health triad. Pets are increasingly used in therapy and social prescribing, dogs are used as support dogs for various disabilities, and animals of course play a key, if contentious, role in research. Production animals are also a significant consideration, and ensuring the health and welfare of these animals can directly affect food system health. There are positive and negative influences and outcomes to the human-animal-environment relationship and the veterinary nurse's role, along with the whole veterinary healthcare team, is to promote and enhance the relationship as much as possible within their scope.

Professionalism and Reflection in Veterinary Nursing, First Edition.
Edited by Sue Badger and Andrea Jeffery.
© 2022 John Wiley & Sons Ltd. Published 2022 by John Wiley & Sons Ltd.
Companion website: www.wiley.com/go/badger/professionalism-veterinary-nursing

Supporting Veterinary Nurses' Well-being

The well-being of the veterinary team and, in this text, that of the veterinary nurse should also never be overlooked. Veterinary nurses experience similar stressors as their veterinary surgeon colleagues, and it is suggested that veterinary nurses are an at-risk group for suffering the effects of occupational stress. Provision of support to others, which is often emotionally and ethically demanding, is a likely contributor in challenging mental health, and research suggests that euthanasia support is a critical occupation-specific stressor which has an impact on veterinary staff (Deacon and Brough 2017).

Communication, Relationship-Building, and Shared Decision-Making

The Value of Effective Communication

The role of the veterinary nurse in primary care and referral practice is expanding. Veterinary nurses have a unique position within the practice team. They have increasing responsibility in clinics and consultations, in client-facing duties such as obtaining informed consent as well as explaining and discussing complex disease conditions, and in end-of-life discussions and euthanasia. It is imperative that veterinary nurses possess the skills to manage these situations confidently and competently, offer clients a positive experience, and maintain the reputation of the profession; proficient communication skills are integral to this.

Regard for the Human-Animal Bond

Whilst the welfare of the animal patient must be the primary consideration for all veterinary professionals as outlined in the Royal College of Veterinary Surgeons' (RCVS's) Code of Professional Conduct for Veterinary Nurses (RCVS 2021), regard and consideration for both the patient *and* the patient's owner or agent, the relationship that exists between them (Figure 5.1), and the three-way interconnection between the healthcare worker, the patient, and the owner, is a consistent theme that runs through all our professional work.

To effectively understand the client's needs and wishes in terms of the patient's treatment, we need to consider and attempt to understand and acknowledge their unique viewpoint, and several of the sections in this chapter will offer examples of how this may be achieved.

Societal Challenges

The greater need for the companionship of pets in modern society, which became increasingly evident during the (c.2020) COVID-19 pandemic, has a potential

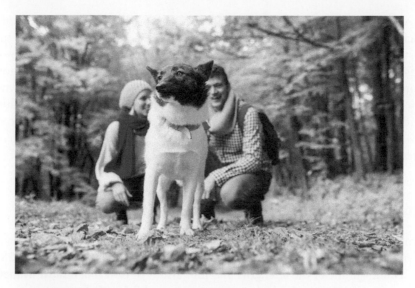

Figure 5.1   The bond between people and their pets is often very strong. Halfpoint/Adobe Stock.

long-term impact on patient welfare. Those who previously had no experience of pet ownership, as well as the acquisition of pets unsuitable for the owner and their circumstances, will undoubtedly unfold over the coming months and years. Behavioural problems developing in puppies and young dogs who received inadequate socialisation or were not habituated to being left alone whilst their owners were working from or at home, will require the support of veterinary and wider professionals. Financial recession may result in many pet owners struggling financially to support adequate healthcare and provide correct husbandry. The financial aspect of veterinary healthcare has always presented a challenge to the profession, and many more pet owners may struggle to meet veterinary fees, leading to difficult ethical decisions over treatment options and euthanasia of treatable animals or those suffering from behavioural issues.

Dog ownership in particular is possibly no longer seen as a privilege but a right, and those in unstable financial and housing situations are acquiring dogs. There is a rise in the breeding and ownership of canine brachycephalic breeds, particularly Pugs (BVA 2018; Packer et al. 2020), despite the work to deter this. Mixed breed 'designer' dogs are on the increase, with novel variants being created at a high rate. The cost of purchasing a dog has risen as demand outweighs supply. Dogs are often utilised to reinforce status and as protectors, and exploited in dog-dog fighting. According to NHS statistics, the increase in injuries from dogs rose by more than 5% between 2015 and 2018, with 23 078 admissions for dog-related injuries between those dates (Royal College of Surgeons of England 2019), suggesting that dogs are in increasingly unsuitable environments, inadequately supervised, and behaviourally mismanaged.

How is the veterinary nurse best placed to support the client given these factors in society? These trends and figures are disheartening; however, they serve to high-light that the role of the veterinary nurse (and the veterinary profession) is to provide education and guidance to clients of pets, whatever their motivation, and to competently handle the legal implications should reporting of pet owners be required due to neglect, cruelty, or illegal activity. Whilst Veterinary Health Care Providers (VHCPs) will have their own views and ethical standpoints, the service offered to clients must attempt to remain non-judgemental in the face of increasing challenges.

Ethical Values

Ethical values also play a part in how veterinary nurses manage difficult ethical challenges and understand client's wishes and actions; Hernandez et al. (2018) offer an excellent outline of the strengths and limitations of differing ethical frameworks. A series of exercises can also be found on the Animal Ethics Dilemma website (www. aedilemma.net), which offers a useful tool for evaluation of ethical perspectives.

Changes in Approach to Communication

The paternalistic approach to healthcare which demonstrates a relationship in which the healthcare professional is the expert who imparts information and makes decisions on behalf of the patient (client) has been replaced in human healthcare over the past two decades by a move towards embodiment of a patient-centred, shared decision-making (SDM) approach, and veterinary medicine is fol-lowing this pathway.

Understanding that clients are often well informed, attempt to seek information elsewhere, play a greater role in administration of care to their pets, and wish to have an input into healthcare decisions; helps us to appreciate why a SDM approach is more beneficial in communication and decision-making with clients.

Compliance, Adherence, and Concordance

The term 'compliance' – the level to which a client has followed given healthcare recommendations – suggests a lack of involvement of the client in this process (Horne et al. 2005). Alternatively, use of the term 'adherence', whilst a related term, can be defined as the degree to which a patient (client) follows agreed recom-mendations. This term places emphasis on agreement (NICE 2007) and there is a discreet yet distinct difference.

Additionally, the concept of 'concordance', which is not a measure of adherence, but refers to the process of incorporating the client's views and wishes in the negotiation on therapeutic decisions (Dickinson et al. 1999; Jordan et al. 2002), encourages VHCPs to build relationships with patients/clients that are based on mutual trust, two-way communication, and empowering the client to have an input to decision-making. This chapter will encompass some of the ways that this can be achieved.

The concept of SDM is also a fundamental part of this equation, and '[t]he main difference between these terms is that shared decision-making terminology encompasses the whole process, whereas concordance is the outcome of that process' (Jordan et al. 2002).

The Importance of Empathy

Empathy is a key factor in effective client communication. Veterinary issues are often complex, emotional, and challenging; with the addition of financial considerations and constraints. Whilst clients often look to us to give practical, technical, and difficult information, empathy is key in helping the client to feel supported and in building trust. All VHCPs perform their role because they care about the welfare of animals and people, and it is vital that this is not lost in the complexities of veterinary or financial discussions.

Whilst some have a natural empathic approach and the ability to demonstrate this, empathy can still be evident in those who may have a more rigid and pragmatic approach to communication.

Ensuring that the client feels heard is a significant factor in empathy. Listening skills may include:

- appropriate eye contact and open body language
- not interrupting
- acknowledging what has been said by the client
- responding to subtle and overt verbal and non-verbal cues
- avoiding thinking about your next question or response (it shows)
- allowing pauses in dialogue to allow the client to think.

Effective listening skills will enable VHCPs to gain far more information from the client and will encourage the client to be open and honest in their information giving, which is invaluable in gaining an accurate history and determining the client's perspective.

Body language is also a vital component of empathy. Use of our own body language, for example; our position in the consulting room and in relation to the client, acknowledgement of and communication with and about the animal, eye contact, touch, facial expressions, tone of voice, and awareness of and responsiveness to client body language – all feed into this (Figure 5.2).

Empathy does not need to be reserved for those more *obvious* situations where we feel it is appropriate, for example in end-of-life discussions; and in fact, it

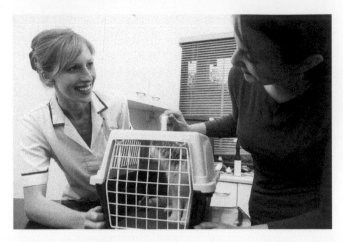

Figure 5.2   Recognising and understanding body language in both pets and their owners is an important skill. Monkey Business/Adobe Stock.

can be useful to employ an empathic approach in many circumstances, for example:

- when desired treatment outcomes are not achieved
- before or during routine procedures such as neutering and nail clips as the patient and/or owner may often be anxious
- discussions surrounding finance, particularly when the client's finances do not stretch to the desired procedure or treatment
- owner difficulty with administering medications, which can be stressful for both parties
- when the client shares difficulties in other, more personal areas of their life
- when clients are upset, frustrated or angry.

The Concept of 'Sharing Information'

When consultation structure is considered, it could be thought that during history-taking we are 'gaining' information from the client. When the treatment options are given, and a treatment plan devised, we may see this as then 'giving' information. However, it is important to view the communication between client and VHCP as a fluid and interchangeable dialogue where information passes both ways throughout the consultation.

In context, if we are offering information regarding a particular treatment, we also need to know from the client whether the treatment aligns with their wishes, is able to be administered, and is affordable. When the client is offering us information on the patient's history or clinical signs, we may need to offer clarity or examples to help them to do this effectively.

It is useful for veterinary nurses to adopt the concept of 'sharing information' as a communication goal during consultations and interactions, and embrace this as a mindset in the approach to all communication with clients, and this is outlined in more detail in recent work to develop a 'Veterinary Nurse-Client Communication Matrix' (Macdonald et al. 2021).

Shared Decision-Making

The practice of SDM is well established in the human healthcare field, with much research completed in this area. The ethical principles which underpin SDM are that clinicians need to support patients to achieve the goal of individual choice, wherever feasible. SDM supports autonomy by building and promoting good relationships between clinicians and patients (in the case of veterinary medicine, between VHCPs and clients), and respecting clients' competence and circumstances (Elwyn et al. 2012).

SDM in the context of veterinary healthcare involves overt inclusion of the pet owner or client in the decision-making process for the animal patient. The processes to achieve this may include:

- highlighting all available treatment options, including risks and benefits
- gaining the client's perspective and views on the options and discussing any concerns
- reaching a mutually agreeable decision on the best option for this particular client and patient, taking their circumstances into consideration.

Veterinary nurses are likely to utilise an SDM approach in many of their interactions with clients, and if we take a simple example such as discussing the most appropriate flea treatment for a patient, then we can see that we need to:

- highlight the available treatments, including method of application, any risk factors, cost and efficacy
- find out about the patient's lifestyle, and what product will best suit this
- ensure that the client is able to apply the treatment
- mutually decide on a treatment based on the discussion, and confirm this decision.

It is important that communication is tailored to the individual, and their communication style and preferences, and current understanding, should be taken into account. Many clients have previous experiences and knowledge (informed clients) and may wish to take a proactive approach in making decisions, whereas other clients may prefer to be guided by the VHCP in decision-making.

Informed Consent

Guidance on informed consent was updated by the RCVS in 2018 (RCVS 2018) and included advice that whilst the most suitable VHCP to gain informed consent is the veterinary surgeon in charge of the case, the responsibility of achieving informed consent may be delegated to a veterinary nurse or student veterinary nurse, providing certain criteria are met (RCVS 2020a).

As in SDM, the term 'informed consent' is self-descriptive – clients must be given the necessary information available to be able to give *informed* consent for any procedure or treatment.

There are potential difficulties in deciding the risk factors for a procedure or treatment that should be disclosed and discussed. Death is a potential outcome of an anaesthetic procedure for example, but clients may not be aware of this unless it is overtly stated. Many drugs or procedures may have potentially devastating side-effects, certain species or breeds of animal are more likely to experience adverse reactions or poor outcomes; and it is the remit of the VHCP to evaluate and decide which information must be given to the client to enable them to make an informed decision, based on the circumstances.

Detailed guidance on the factors in successfully gaining informed consent can be accessed within the Code of Professional Conduct (RCVS 2020a), and includes consideration of:

- the relationship of the client to the animal (for example, owner or agent)
- the factors that should be considered during the consent discussion
- the VHCP most appropriate for being responsible for gaining the consent
- consent forms
- discussion of fees
- public health
- young people and children
- mental incapacity
- wildlife.

It is vital that any VHCP who has responsibility for gaining consent is aware of and follows this guidance.

Motivational Interviewing

Motivational interviewing is a client-centred, relationship-based approach, originally developed in the 1980s by Rollnick and Miller for discussions with patients suffering drug addiction and alcohol abuse, to elicit change behaviour. The technique has not yet been fully explored within the veterinary profession, although one study performed by Bard et al. (2017) demonstrated encouraging results.

The technique of motivational interviewing is worthy of mention since the principles are of great benefit to the veterinary nurse when discussing treatment options or disease management with clients. It has particular relevance in many of the scenarios that veterinary nurses manage, such as weight and chronic disease management, where motivation and commitment of the client is imperative.

In motivational interviewing in the context of veterinary consultations, the VHCP aims to identify the motivators that the client may hold in affecting change through following a treatment plan or adhering to a programme. If we consider a

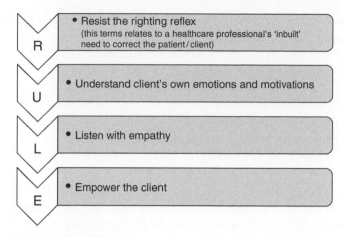

R • Resist the righting reflex
(this terms relates to a healthcare professional's 'inbuilt' need to correct the patient/client)

U • Understand client's own emotions and motivations

L • Listen with empathy

E • Empower the client

Figure 5.3   The RULE acronym.

weight management consultation, it can be natural for the VHCP, in understanding the welfare implications for obesity, to impress on the client that the animal *must* lose weight; that the client's actions in overfeeding their pet are having a negative impact on the patient. This creates immediate conflict in communication, where the client will seek reasons why this has happened and why calorie restriction and weight loss are not possible. By identifying reasons why the client themselves may wish the pet to lose weight – for example by asking about how the animal used to be prior to becoming obese, what things they are no longer able to do, how it makes the client feel (referred to as 'eliciting change talk') – we are working *with* the client in creating a positive and proactive mindset, rather than laying blame or dictating recommendations that the client may not be motivated to follow.

The technique is not simple to become proficient in and may take several training sessions with the inclusion of detailed feedback (Schwalbe et al. 2014); however, the overarching principles are an excellent starting point.

The key principles are:

1. *Engage* the client in talking about the issues, gain their perspective and trust.
2. *Focus* on finding out the factors that the client may wish to change or achieve.
3. *Evoke* the reasons behind why the client may want to make the change.
4. *Plan* with the client, an aim that will be achievable for them and their pet.

We can also use the RULE acronym for further basic guidance, see Figure 5.3.

Now look at Exercise 5.1 in the additional resources for this chapter (www. wiley.com/go/badger/professionalism-veterinary-nursing).

Consultation Structure

Structure in a veterinary consultation provides a clear framework to guide the VHCP in organising the consultation and will assist the client in giving and assimilating information. In general, all consultations or discussions follow a typical format: planning and preparation, opening the consultation or discussion, sharing of information (gathering information [± clinical examination] and giving information) and closing the consultation or discussion.

Providing structure to a consultation:

- offers a professional approach
- assists with time management
- helps to ensure that nothing is missed
- provides assurance to the client.

Whilst consultations differ greatly in terms of their focus (from a routine vaccination to an emergency consultation for example), use of a framework is applicable and beneficial in applying structure to all discussions with clients.

Currently, the most utilised framework for veterinary communication is the Guide to the Veterinary Consultation based on the Calgary Cambridge Model (GVCCCM) (Radford et al. 2006) which outlines a seven-step process in approaching consultations and includes supplementary guidance to support the framework (Figure 5.4).

An outline of the GVCCCM is shown in Figure 5.4, which includes additional guidance points for each stage of the consultation.

The Veterinary Nurse-Client Communication Matrix (Macdonald et al. 2021) is the result of research to develop a veterinary nurse-specific guide to client communication and offers an outline graphic, which is cyclical in nature, incorporating a reflective practice component. Further detail on all elements of communication skills specific to veterinary nurses are expanded on in the full Matrix (Figure 5.5).

Managing Conflict

During situations that involve conflict or grievance, communication can become more challenging, and it takes practice and confidence to be able to handle difficult situations effectively. Many conflicts arise due to previous breakdown in communication, emotionally charged situations, and financial disagreements. It is imperative that we first and foremost remember that these situations can be difficult for our clients, and our duty is to help to resolve them, despite often feeling that they are unjustified or unfair. Empathy is a key diffuser in handing conflict. Stepping away from a public area, listening to the client's grievance and trying to appreciate their perspective, ensuring that you have the correct information, and empathising with the situation are the first steps in reaching resolution. Once the problem is understood, then the VHCP can work towards a mutual resolution with the client.

Our own and others' safety is of course paramount, and every practice should have a protocol for managing conflict situations which escalate.

When a situation has evolved where an error has been made, or a sequence of events has led to a negative situation; demonstrating the steps that the practice has taken to prevent this recurring can provide further reassurance to the client.

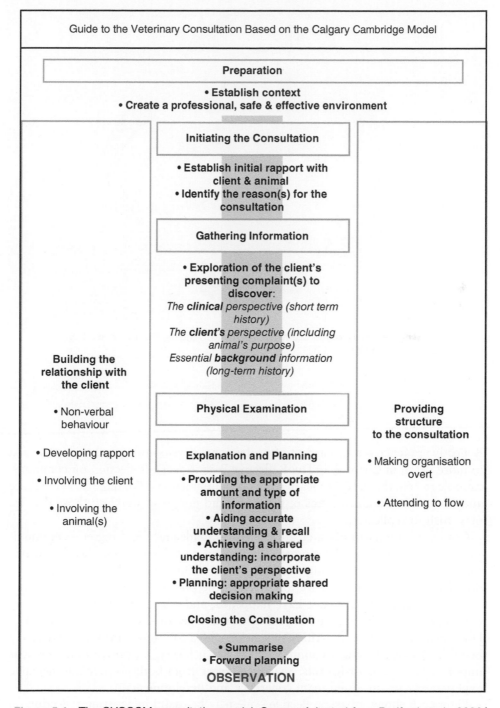

Guide to the Veterinary Consultation Based on the Calgary Cambridge Model

Preparation

- **Establish context**
- **Create a professional, safe & effective environment**

Initiating the Consultation

- **Establish initial rapport with client & animal**
- **Identify the reason(s) for the consultation**

Gathering Information

- **Exploration of the client's presenting complaint(s) to discover:**
The **clinical** perspective (short term history)
The **client's** perspective (including animal's purpose)
Essential **background** information (long-term history)

Physical Examination

Explanation and Planning

- **Providing the appropriate amount and type of information**
- **Aiding accurate understanding & recall**
- **Achieving a shared understanding: incorporate the client's perspective**
- **Planning: appropriate shared decision making**

Closing the Consultation

- **Summarise**
- **Forward planning**
OBSERVATION

Building the relationship with the client

- Non-verbal behaviour
- Developing rapport
- Involving the client
- Involving the animal(s)

Providing structure to the consultation

- Making organisation overt
- Attending to flow

Figure 5.4   The GVCCCM consultation model. Source: Adapted from Radford et al., 2006/ AAVMC.

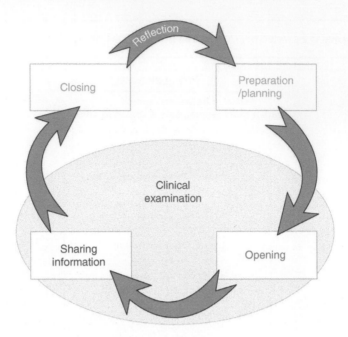

Figure 5.5   The veterinary nurse client communication matrix. Source: Based on Macdonald, Gray and Robbé, 2021.

Reflective Practice in Relation to Development of Communication Skills

Reflective practice is a key aspect of professional development, and this is covered in more detail in Chapter 8 (The Reflective Practitioner). Reflection on communication can help the VHCP to learn from client interactions (Fontaine 2018; Wallace and May 2016), both in terms of those that did not go so well and those that we may wish to replicate.

Communication can often create feelings of inadequacy and regret – communication is very much 'in the moment' with often no time to think ahead, and this can create distress when things haven't gone well and we are left with feelings of doubt and self-criticism. Reflection gives us the processing space to think about what happened, why it might have happened, and what we could do differently next time; ultimately it can aid in professional and personal well-being (May 2017). Documenting reflection in writing or sharing with a colleague can also be extremely helpful. Conversely, when communication has achieved a positive outcome, it is important to acknowledge this. Sharing learning from both positive and negative experiences can also build team coherence and development.

Figure 5.6 shows a basic reflective cycle may be useful in assisting reflection on a communication experience.

Now look at Exercise 5.2 in the additional resources for this chapter (www.wiley.com/go/badger/professionalism-veterinary-nursing).

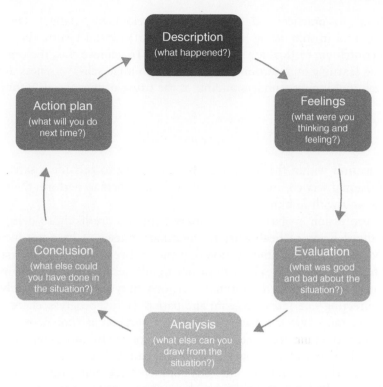

Figure 5.6   Adapted from Gibbs' 1988 reflective model. Source: Adapted from Gibbs 1988.

A Just, Learning Culture

Supporting a culture of openness regarding reporting of adverse incidents offers staff more confidence in sharing mistakes, provides support for staff well-being and emotional health, and facilitates learning which can be shared with the wider team. This is often referred to as a 'just culture' or 'no-blame culture'. Much research has been performed in this area in human healthcare, in terms of both patient safety and staff well-being. However, 'just culture' does not simply mean a blame-free culture, but rather a culture of 'balanced accountability' (Paradiso and Sweeney 2019), and examination of the organisational processes which may have led to the error. It asks 'what' is the cause of the error, rather than 'who' (Oxtoby 2017).

A culture of learning works synergistically with areas of development such as clinical audit and quality improvement, allowing events to be explored in an open and non-judgemental setting.

Veterinary workplaces should ensure that a just and learning organisational culture is overtly embraced and encouraged, and that all staff understand the principles. If staff members are confident that an appropriate balance will be used when dealing with accountability and errors, that sharing learning from mistakes is beneficial to practice and professional development, patient safety, client experience, and in supporting and promoting staff mental health, they are more likely to contribute to this in a positive manner. To achieve this, the organisation must value learning and accountability, and encourage self-awareness and reflection, which will improve understanding of the cause of mistakes (Oxtoby 2018).

The Importance of Team Communication

Communication within the team must be exemplary to provide a safe, effective, and professional service, and to enable all team members to perform their function effectively and with fulfilment.

As the profession evolves and veterinary surgeons are likely to delegate more tasks in the delivery of healthcare to veterinary nurses, it becomes increasingly imperative that a clear communication sequence between parties is understood and adhered to. Veterinary nurses have the scope to take responsibility for many aspects of patient care. However, the ultimate responsibility for the patient always lies with the directing veterinary surgeon; and patient status, progress, client concerns, or any issues must be relayed to the veterinary surgeon as soon as is possible. In the consultation setting, it is useful to develop a strategy for managing this, whether it be through a written summary of patients handled that day, or via a verbal discussion. In the hospital or clinic environment, managing this through ward-rounds, where relevant staff involved in the patients' care are present, is an effective method for ensuring that communication of issues, plans, and progress takes place; and the veterinary nurse should be empowered to have a significant contribution in this process and be involved in clinical decision-making regarding the patient.

When patient care is transferred to other staff, there should be a clear handover process, including both the patient's status and care and the communication that has taken place with the client, to provide effective continuity of care (Kerrigan 2020).

Client wishes or any situation which impacts on the patient's care should be clearly stated, on clinical records and verbally, to those involved in the delivery of care. These wishes may have originated from any team member, including receptionist and support staff, so practices should have a policy for ensuring that all necessary team members are informed.

Daily 'huddles' - short meetings at the start of the day or at the start of each shift (Institute for Healthcare Improvement n.d.), and regular team meetings (Figure 5.7) also have an impact on communication within the team, and enhancement of the service offered to clients.

The Veterinary Nurse's Role as Client Advocate

Chapter 4 addresses many of the factors involved in addressing clinical advocacy. In this section, we will explore the communication concepts that enhance advocacy from the client's perspective.

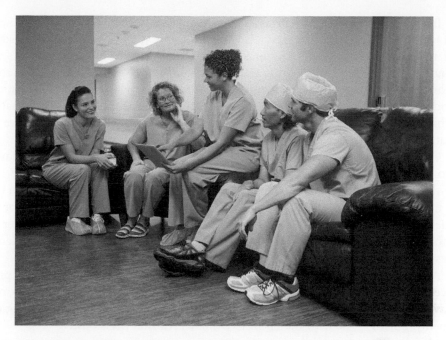

Figure 5.7   Regular team meetings are important elements of the working day. Tyler Olson/ Adobe Stock.

The duties of the veterinary nurse in meeting both the needs of the patient and of the client may often present conflict. In accordance with the professional responsibilities as outlined in the Code of Conduct for Veterinary Nurses, 'Veterinary nurses must make animal health and welfare their first consideration when attending to animals' (RCVS 2020a), however there may be situations where this does not align with the client's wishes, for example in delaying euthanasia or in declining treatment.

Gaining and Understanding the Animal Owner's Perspective

Understanding of the human-animal bond and the client's relationship with the animal affects every unique situation we may encounter, and the relationships that veterinary nurses develop with clients and their animals often offer a deeper insight into this. Clients may be more candid with veterinary nurses about their goals and desires, ethical concerns, personal and financial circumstances, and ability to administer treatment, which potentially feed into what may be achievable in terms of treatment and outcome for any particular patient. Ensuring that the client's perspective is sought and listened to without judgement, and that they are helped to communicate in treatment decision-making, is a fundamental principle of advocacy.

Offering the client information on the expectations with regard to outcomes, complications, and cost; and reaching mutual agreement through a SDM process, enables the client to be part of the process.

Being clear about the patient welfare consequences of client decisions is also part of the veterinary nurse's role, but it is vital that this is approached from the position of understanding and appreciation of the client's perspective, even if it does not align with our own views, values, and professional responsibilities. This does create ethical conflict when the client's wishes do not meet the welfare needs of the patient, and the VHCP's role is to negotiate the situation empathically, offer information which can assist the client in understanding the implications, and achieve an outcome that both parties agree on, despite their differing perspectives.

Clients are increasingly well informed, and many clients will seek information from beyond the veterinary practice on their pet's condition. This of course brings with it some challenges, since there is an abundance of inaccurate information that is not based on current available evidence. However, we should offer credit for the client's diligence in performing research, and question as a profession whether we should contribute to more readily accessible, accurate, unbiased, and evidence-based information (Belshaw 2018).

Advances in human medicine, and televised documentaries of veterinary practice, often highlighting complex procedures but omitting the cost implications, may have an influence on client expectations. The role of the VHCP is to explore options openly, but to work with the client to come to realistic decisions.

Assisting the Client to Communicate their Views

Whilst it is the role of the veterinary surgeon to make final treatment decisions with the client, the veterinary nurse can play a key role in assisting with the communication process. It might be that the client wishes the nurse to have those discussions directly, but often a pre-arranged consultation where the client is able to offer their input assisted by support from the veterinary nurse will be appropriate in facilitating an effective decision-making process.

Veterinary nurses can support this by:

- helping clients to source further information that is at a level appropriate to any previous knowledge and their cognitive abilities
- helping clients to involve other stakeholders (for example family members)
- assisting in finding solutions to problems, such as transport, administration of medicines, client disabilities affecting patient care
- writing down any concerns and thoughts and creating a plan for approaching the discussion.

The Value of Nurse-Led Consultations in Supporting Owners

The trend suggests that veterinary nurses are performing an increasing number of nurse-led clinics and consultations in the UK (Robinson 2019), and the veterinary nursing profession aspires to clients viewing veterinary nurses as an important contributor to the ongoing health of their animals and a valuable source of

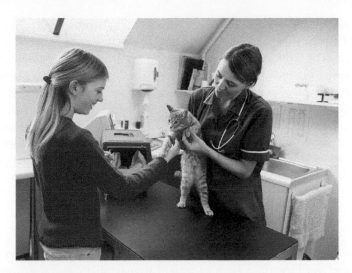

Figure 5.8   Nurse clinics are now a normal part of practice life. Monkey Business/Adobe Stock.

information and guidance. As part of the vet-led team and under the direction of a veterinary surgeon, veterinary nurses are ideally positioned to provide healthcare advice and support on many levels – from preventative healthcare to acute injury, chronic disease management and end-of-life care. The veterinary nursing qualification in the UK facilitates the knowledge and competence to manage these types of consultations; specific professional development in key areas increases the level of expertise that nurses can share with clients, and further enhances the confidence in veterinary surgeons to delegate this work.

Clients may find nurses easier to talk to about ongoing concerns with pet healthcare and behavioural management and will seek advice from nurses, following a consultation and during treatment, to fill in knowledge gaps, seek reassurance, or clarify information (Figure 5.8). They may feel that the veterinary surgeon's time is scarce and that consultations are strictly time-limited, but that nurses have more space to devote to such conversations, and perhaps more perception of and empathy with the client's concerns, and the relationship that exists between the patient and the owner. Evolvement of the human healthcare model, with increasing prevalence of nurse practitioners being responsible for tasks and duties that previously only doctors carried out, may also have an influence on how the public views veterinary nurses and the level of healthcare support they are able to provide as our profession also evolves.

Advances in our Profession

In the UK, the VN Futures Project (www.vnfutures.org.uk) aims to clarify and address the challenges the veterinary nursing profession faces, and exploit the opportunities available to enable progression. One of the ambitions of the project is to achieve 'A clarified and bolstered VN role via a reformed Schedule 3' (VN Futures 2016), thus expanding the role of the veterinary nurse through potential legislative reform. Following work to develop a delegation framework to assist veterinary surgeons and nurses in the process, the RCVS Legislative Working Party was formed, and a report of proposed changes was approved by the RCVS Council in July 2020 (RCVS 2020b). Consultation with the professions and public was held during early 2021, and the work will be reviewed by the Department for Environment, Food and Rural Affairs (Defra). Any legislative reform is a slow process; however, this process is essential to ensure that all relevant parties have been consulted prior to parliamentary debate and legislative change.

Preventative Healthcare Consultations

Preventative healthcare consultations may include start-of-life, adolescent, particular healthcare considerations such as weight management and nutrition, and geriatric patient care.

The veterinary profession gives a great deal of consideration to preventative healthcare in the long-term management of animal health and welfare and the veterinary nurse's role within this. The veterinary nurse should be viewed as the cornerstone in these healthcare contact-points.

It is now commonplace for the second part of a primary vaccination to be administered by a veterinary nurse, and nurses having sufficient time allocated to discuss the multi-factorial nature of animal care and health is vital, but it is also valuable to promote regular check-ups with the nurse throughout the pet's development phase.

Routine preventative measures, such as parasite control, correct nutrition, exercise and environment, and behavioural issues; and their value in ensuring the health of the nation's pets cannot be underestimated. The veterinary nurse can offer information, guidance, and support in ensuring that the most appropriate options are selected; and this takes effective communication with the client to ensure their needs and specific situations are factored into the decisions.

Geriatric patients of all species require monitoring for development of disease conditions, with intervention under the direction of a veterinary surgeon when necessary. It is of benefit for the geriatric patient to receive ongoing healthcare examinations as their age advances, with relevant advice given to their guardians to ensure that their needs are met in order to promote welfare and quality of life. Owners may be reticent to seek advice on conditions in older pets, often fearing traumatic outcomes or financial costs that they are unable to meet. Establishing an ongoing healthcare routine and relationship with the client and patient will embolden the client to more readily consult the practice with any concerns.

The Role of the Veterinary Nurse in Long-Term Disease Management

Current data suggests that the care of patients suffering from chronic disease is not significantly supported by nurse-led clinics (Robinson 2019). The historical

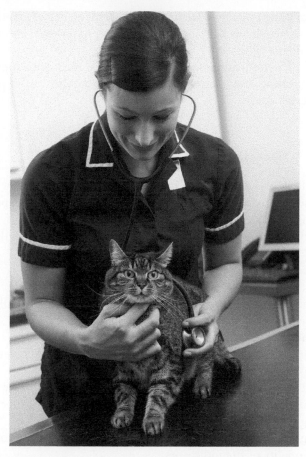

Figure 5.9   The RVN can play a vital role in supporting the owners of pets with long-term illnesses. Monkey Business/Adobe Stock.

approach has been for veterinary surgeons to manage these patients, with regular consultations to assess progress and direct diagnostics and treatment. The utilisation of veterinary nurses to provide ongoing healthcare in a significant proportion of chronic disease patients could markedly increase over the coming years, due to a variety of factors (Figure 5.9):

- veterinary nurses wishing to have a more significant role in managing such patients
- increased expertise levels of veterinary nurses, through focused professional development and training
- the Certificate in Advanced Veterinary Nursing leading to nurses being able to specialise in particular areas of patient care
- increased confidence in veterinary surgeons to delegate ongoing care of such patients
- developments in practice culture, embracing a 'vet-led team' approach
- the profession acknowledging the need for veterinary nurses to have greater role satisfaction through delegation and increased responsibility and recognition

- clients' increasing acknowledgement of the competence of veterinary nurses
- a shortage of veterinary surgeons, necessitating more efficient utilisation of the veterinary nurses' skillset
- financial difficulties leading to reduced available income to spend on pets, and veterinary nursing consultations having the flexibility to be placed within a lower price-bracket.

Potential Impact

The level of support that could be offered to clients in managing their pets with chronic disease could have a substantial impact on the client's experience, success with managing treatment and, ultimately, patient outcomes. If we consider a disease condition such as osteoarthritis, the role of the nurse could involve areas such as:

- helping clients fully understand the disease process
- giving information on the range of drugs and supplements available
- ensuring any weight management issues are addressed
- offering guidance on exercise and nutrition
- performing a house visit and addressing environmental issues such as steps, stairs, slippery floors, access to vehicles
- offering basic physiotherapy, stretching and strength-building exercises
- taking regular blood samples to monitor hepatic and renal function
- performing radiography
- performing pain scoring assessments and helping the client to do this at home
- discussing quality of life indicators.

Whilst these areas can be addressed during a veterinary consultation, many patients with osteoarthritis may only visit the practice at three-monthly or longer intervals, usually for check-up for repeat prescription of analgesic drugs, for example. Engaging the client in a long-term programme allows for more detailed discussion of the components of disease management, facilitating factors to be addressed that may otherwise not have been. It offers the client an ongoing and regular connection with the practice, ensures that clinical deterioration and improvement are monitored, and builds a relationship between the veterinary nurse, the client and the patient.

The Vet-Led Team

The concept of the vet-led team amplifies the ethos of delivery of care through a multi-professional approach, utilising the differing skills, attributes, and areas of expertise available within the profession to provide the best possible healthcare and client support.

The British Veterinary Association (BVA), in their 2019 policy statement on the vet-led team, used the analogy of a 'hub and spoke' as a model for provision of veterinary care, with the veterinary surgeon being the central hub, directing clients to the additional services offered by trained veterinary professionals, including veterinary nurses (BVA 2019). The scope of the model incorporates a wide variety of additional veterinary allied professionals, for example, veterinary physiotherapists and hydrotherapists, equine dental technicians, foot trimmers, meat hygiene inspectors, groomers, animal behaviourists, and animal care assistants.

The model allows us to visualise a profession whereby the veterinary surgeon is central to decision-making, but the profession gains strength and works most effectively as a whole, with contributions from a variety of allied professionals. Within veterinary practice in the provision of day-to-day healthcare to patients and their owners, veterinary nurses will be the professionals that veterinary surgeons most often direct and delegate to.

The BVA cites the overarching benefits of the model as being:

- better animal health, animal welfare and public health outcomes
- improved client care
- provision of more integrated animal care
- improved clinical provision or assurance on food hygiene controls
- more effective and efficient use of skills within the veterinary professions
- a strengthened veterinary workforce, with the potential to ease capacity concerns and difficulties recruiting and retaining both vets and RVNs
- improved well-being for veterinary surgeons, RVNs, and allied professionals
- more sustainable veterinary businesses.

(BVA, 2019)

The RCVS, through the work of the Legislation Working Party, incorporated recommendations within their 2020 Report on the regulation of veterinary paraprofessionals, which would enable a regulatory framework incorporating allied professionals to be developed (Cox 2020; May 2020).

The District or Community Veterinary Nurse Role

In promoting the values of the provision of client support throughout an animal's life, and veterinary healthcare to populations who are unable or have difficulty in accessing practice premises, the concept of district or community veterinary nursing has a strong supporting argument. Pet owners may have obstacles preventing them bringing their pet to the practice such as disabilities which make it difficult to monitor and medicate animals, and certainly some animals are averse to, and stressed within, the practice environment. In addition, nurses performing visits within the client's home could have an enormous value in both palliative and end-of-life care (Kerrigan 2014), in terms of both the client and patient experience, and the viability of providing this service.

District nursing within human healthcare has been developing since its origins in 1859 (QNI 2009), and is a highly valuable aspect of human healthcare provision. The Royal College of Nursing recognises that district nurses have a higher level of autonomy and must develop strong decision-making capabilities to perform their role effectively. The National Health Service also provides clear and structured safety and safeguarding guidelines for district nurses due to the lone nature of the work, increased pressures, and visiting potentially vulnerable patients.

The core values, beliefs, and challenges of district nursing, which would also be applicable to a veterinary district nurse role, include:

- keeping patients at home where they want to be
- the relationship between nurse and patient (and client)
- preventative and supportive role
- unpredictable and changeable role, requiring nurses to be responsive, flexible and adaptable
- responsive and proactive in managing both long and short-term patients and conditions
- autonomous, yet highly dependent on other healthcare professionals
- difficulties with leadership opportunities and career structure, and lack of recognition of this specialised role
- recognition of the significant difference between nursing in the clinical environment; and nursing in patients' homes; each require different skills, training, aptitude and leadership.

(adapted from The Queen's Nursing Institute, 2009)

It is recognised that many veterinary practices already deliver certain veterinary nursing services within client's homes; however, there is currently no educational framework for district veterinary nursing, or a profession-wide safety and safeguarding policy. Advances in the profession could potentially develop the role with reference to the model followed in human healthcare.

Legislation currently dictates that veterinary nursing work must be directed by a veterinary surgeon, and that the nurse must also be working in the employment of the veterinary surgeon (or an employer whom the veterinary surgeon is representing). This therefore prohibits district nurses from working on a freelance basis, with a client base from several different local practices, and limits the work to the practice that the nurse is employed by. One of the proposals in the RCVS Legislation Working Party's Report (RCVS 2020b) suggests the 'uncoupling' of direction from employment, which would provide a greater level of flexibility in functionality of the service; however, there are considerations that need to be made to ensure that the work of veterinary nurses remains genuinely vet-led (BVA 2021).

Palliative Care

Palliative care is the supportive care of patients starting from any point that they are diagnosed with a life-threatening or terminal disease, and the objective of

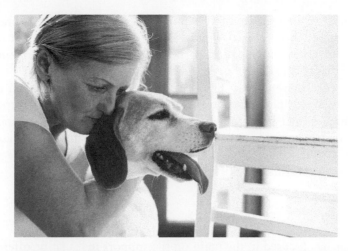

Figure 5.10   The RVN is ideally placed to provide appropriate support for the palliative case. Halfpoint/Adobe Stock.

palliative care is to maintain or improve the quality of life for patients and support their owners (Figure 5.10) (World Health Organisation 2020). It is important to remember that 'terminal' may include a variety of disease conditions such as osteo-arthritis, cardiac disease or renal disease, as well as disease conditions such as neoplasia, which many clients may instantly conclude is a life-ending illness. There is a distinction between palliative and hospice care, which is highlighted later in the chapter.

There are of course many factors involved in this process, including helping pet owners to come to terms with the inevitable loss of their pet, relief from pain, suffering and other problems associated with their disease condition. In addition the nurse will provide support to enable the pet to live as full a life as possible within the timeframe, and offer support during therapies or diagnostics. Palliative care can only effectively be achieved through a vet-led team approach, but there is an undeniable contribution that the veterinary nurse can make to this aspect of patient care.

Following diagnosis of life-threatening disease, the veterinary nurse can offer ongoing structure and support to the client through coordination of a clear disease management plan, including pain assessment and management, nutritional support advice, exercise, and enrichment, delivered through face-to-face, remote, or home consultations at regular intervals. Models such as the HHHHHMM scale (Villalobos 2008) can be used to assist VHCPs and owners to assess quality of life on an ongoing basis.

Veterinary nurses are also ideally placed for the provision of the emotional support that owners of terminally ill patients will need, and there are an increasing number of learning opportunities for nurses wishing to understand more in this area.

Discussing and planning the end-of-life stage for a pet will enable the owner to understand the options available and have an input to this process, offering them a higher degree of control and autonomy. Whilst this is a difficult conversation to have, there are far greater benefits for the client to have time to consider what they would prefer for their pet and to assimilate the information at a time when they are able to make more objective judgements, include the wishes of other family members, and access information to help them with decision-making than, for example, if this is considered at the point of euthanasia.

Palliative care in veterinary practice, delivered in a planned and constructive format, is a relatively new concept. However, with the increasingly recognised value of the human-animal bond, and with advances in veterinary medicine meaning that more treatment options are available for life-threatening disease in animal patients, it is likely that this area of medicine will become far more prevalent in the veterinary profession (Goldberg 2016).

Ongoing Support Including Follow-Up and Telephone Support

This chapter has focused in the main on the support that can be offered to clients by veterinary nurses during face-to-face consultations. However, there is a very strong position for providing both telephone and remote support to clients. A phone call the day after a procedure, and prior to the post-operative (attended) consultation, can help to ascertain any difficulties the patient or client has experienced, whether the patient is eating, drinking and toileting, address any pain management concerns, and so on. This provides the client with a clear connection to healthcare support and assists in identifying and addressing any problems that may otherwise not have been highlighted until the next appointment.

Follow-up calls can also be useful in assessing patient progress in many other disease conditions; again, providing a point of contact and reassurance that the veterinary nurse is available to offer any assistance if required (Figure 5.11).

Communication via the telephone can be more challenging, since the non-verbal communication that can be conveyed in person is unavailable to both parties. We are therefore unable to demonstrate non-verbal communication or visualise and act upon non-verbal cues from the client. Tone of voice that reflects the gravity of

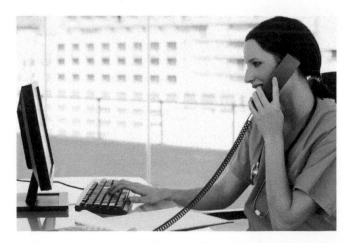

Figure 5.11   Effective follow-up and telephone support are an essential part of the RVN's armoury. WavebreakmediaMicro/Adobe Stock.

the matter being discussed, use of pauses, and noises to acknowledge listening, are therefore vital in these conversations. Use of video calls can help to overcome some of these difficulties, and will also enable us to visualise the patient, but it's important that the client (and the VHCP) is comfortable using, and has access to, the software necessary to facilitate this.

The Role of Veterinary Nurses in Provision of End-of-Life Care

Palliative and end-of-life (hospice) care are terms that are often used interchangeably. However, there is a distinction between these terms. As outlined earlier, palliative care is the supportive care of patients starting from any point that they are diagnosed with a life-threatening or terminal disease, whereas hospice or end-of-life care denotes the care given to patients during the final stages of their life (Kerrigan 2013).

As discussed in a previous section, the provision of palliative care to veterinary patients is an extremely valuable part of the end-of-life process, enabling veterinary professionals to maintain or enhance the quality of life of patients with a terminal illness. Hospice care provides an extension of palliative care, where the goal should be to achieve the best quality of life possible, alongside supporting clients to make the decisions that are in the best interests of their pet, including at their end-of-life. It is imperative that clients understand that neither palliative nor hospice care is an alternative to euthanasia, but exists to support the patient until euthanasia becomes necessary (Kerrigan 2013).

Hospice care has the potential to be an extremely emotionally challenging period, particularly for the pet owner, but also for the VHCP providing the support. In caring for patients and their owners during this time, VHCPs and clients are likely to build closer relationships, which whilst of benefit in SDM and assisting and emotionally supporting the client, will also present a considerable emotional challenge for the VHCP. It is therefore vital that if hospice care is to be undertaken, VHCPs are provided with access to informal and formal support structures.

Whilst hospice care is not yet prevalent in the UK veterinary profession, there has been development of dedicated teams who provide palliative, hospice, and end-of life care within client's homes (www.dignipets.co.uk).

The benefits of hospice care can of course be extremely significant to pet owners who face the loss of their pet, by giving them the option to provide supported care for their pet during the most difficult and upsetting stage of their life and in giving them the reassurance that they have done the very best for them.

End-of-Life Planning

Provision of end-of-life, euthanasia planning can provide the client with the understanding of what will happen to their pet at the end of their life and enable them to have an input to this process. The common current approach to veterinary euthanasia is for the discussion regarding what will happen, how it will happen, and decisions such as cremation options; to occur at the time the pet is brought into the clinic for euthanasia. During this extremely difficult and emotionally challenging consultation, the client is already likely to be overwhelmed by the situation and very unlikely to be able to, or wish to, process this information, and may make decisions that they later regret. This planning can be incorporated as part of palliative or hospice care, or as a distinct appointment, either at home or in the practice.

Very much in the way that people will often outline their burial preferences, what song they would like played at their funeral, and which picture they would like to appear on their order-of-service, pet owners appreciate the opportunity to think ahead and make decisions with the benefit of time and composure.

Veterinary nurses will probably have already built a strong and trusting relationship with the client and their pet, making them ideally placed to offer support during this discussion. It is not an easy undertaking however, and nurses should have been given training and support to enable them to deliver this service confidently and empathically. It is vital that veterinary nurses are also provided with the means to obtain support following difficult conversations and euthanasia procedures.

Support of Animal Owners During and Beyond End-of-Life (Euthanasia) Consultations

Euthanasia appointments should be allocated sufficient time to ensure the client does not feel rushed. The veterinary nurse can spend time with the client and their pet, before and after euthanasia so that they feel supported. Pet owners often wish to reflect on their pet's life and share happy memories, and time should be taken to listen and share their recollections.

It is important to pay regard to the client's wishes where possible; for example, it may be that they want other family members to be present, or they may wish for the pet's collar or a particular blanket to stay with them after euthanasia.

Empathy has been highlighted in a previous section of this chapter and, of course, empathy and understanding towards the client is without doubt the most significant communication skill that we can demonstrate at a pet's end-of-life.

Creating an Appropriate Environment for Euthanasia Appointments

Practices are now commonly meeting the needs of clients during euthanasia appointments, with provision of separate rooms set up for this purpose. These rooms provide a more appropriate environment than the harshness of the clinical consultation room, and several considerations can be made when setting up the room, such as:

- a quiet room, preferably away from other consulting rooms
- quiet closure on the room door
- lower lighting level and soft colour scheme
- soft chairs and/or sofa
- the availability of clean rugs and blankets

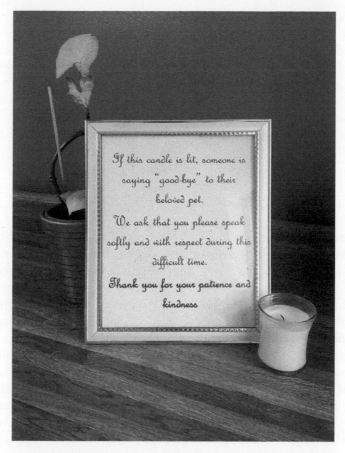

Figure 5.12 Sensitive management of end of life situations within the veterinary practice must be a priority. Battle Ground Veterinary Clinic.

- flowers, or objects which soften the feel of the room
- tissues and wastepaper bin
- immediate access to the necessary paperwork and clinical items required for the appointment
- the ability for the client to leave by an alternative exit to the waiting room.

An idea which has been adopted by many practices is the use of an electric candle in the waiting room to signpost to other clients that a euthanasia appointment is taking place so that they are aware and able demonstrate respect and empathy (Figure 5.12).

Bereavement

The loss of a pet can be an incredibly difficult emotional experience for the pet owner, and clients can experience a similar grief process, sense of loss and psychological impact to that felt at the loss of a human companion (Hewson 2014).

It is difficult to clarify the level of support that should be offered by veterinary practices to clients following the loss of their pet. Many veterinary staff may not have specific training in grief and bereavement counselling, and therefore the means to effectively support the complex grief process. Clients can be signposted to sources of further support, and practices can obtain written information to give to clients to access in their own time. It is important to consider that many clients may not outwardly demonstrate grief or the need for support, and we should offer signposting to help and support to all clients who have suffered the loss of a pet (Hewson 2014).

The Emotional Impact on VHCPs

It is recognised that there are likely to be effects on the mental well-being of veterinary nurses from assisting with euthanasia and supporting clients during euthanasia and bereavement, and if the appropriate support is not provided for the VHCP, this may result in compassion fatigue (Hewson 2015). Veterinary organisations should demonstrate responsibility for the care of staff through the availability of both informal, intra-professional support, and in having a formal support structure in place ready to provide additional care to those staff who require it. It is also vital that management or supervisory staff have received training to enable them to detect signs of stress in their staff (Figure 5.13).

The final stages of a pet's life are often cited by pet owners as being the most harrowing and emotionally difficult time of their life. The support, empathy, and understanding that veterinary nurses can offer to clients during this time, and the value that this will hold for the client and their pet, is something that most veterinary

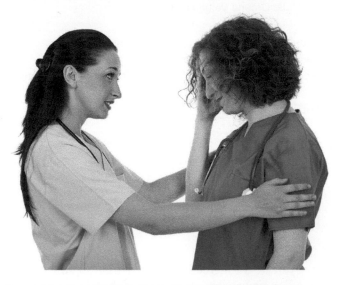

Figure 5.13   Support for the veterinary team. Gabriel Blaj/Adobe Stock.

nurses hold dear, despite the huge responsibility that it carries. Being there for the client and their pet is the reason we perform this role, and it is something in which veterinary nurses take great pride.

Final Thoughts

Thus the support that veterinary nurses provide for the pet owner and patient goes full cycle. From the client bringing a pet to the practice for their first appointment, guiding them through the early and adolescent stages of their life, right through to caring for them through their senior years and sharing their final moments.

It is such an immense privilege to be a part of our clients' and patients' lives; to be afforded the opportunity to have such an impact, and to use our knowledge, skills, care, and kindness to make such a significant difference and to help our clients negotiate care of their pet throughout their life cycle. Whilst this brings with it emotional challenge, most veterinary nurses would not change it for the world.

References

Bard, A.M., Main, D.C.J., Haase, A.M. et al. (2017). The future of veterinary communication: partnership or persuasion? A qualitative investigation of veterinary communication in the pursuit of client behaviour change. *PLoS One* 12 (3): e0171380. https://doi.org/10.1371/journal.pone.0171380.

Belshaw, Z. (2018). Why is Dr Google so popular, and should vets be worried? https://hillsglobalsymposium.com/why-is-dr-google-so-popular-and-should-vets-be-worried-zoe-belshaw (accessed 6 January 2022).

British Veterinary Association. (2018). Our policies. Brachycephalic dogs. https://www.bva.co.uk/take-action/our-policies/brachycephalic-dogs (accessed 6 January 2022).

Cox, L. (2020). LWP update 2: paraprofessional regulation. *Vet. Rec.* 187 (2): 54–55. https://doi.org/10.1136/vr.m2955.

Deacon, R. and Brough, P. (2017). Veterinary nurses' psychological well-being: the impact of patient suffering and death. *Aust. J. Psychol.* 69 (2): 77–85. https://doi.org/10.1111/ajpy.12119.

Dickinson, D., Wilkie, P., and Harris, M. (1999). Taking medicines: concordance is not compliance. *Br. Med. J. (Clin. Res. Ed.)* 319 (7212): 787. https://doi.org/10.1136/bmj.319.7212.787.

Elwyn, G., Frosch, D., Thomson, R., Joseph-Williams, N., et al. (2012) 'Shared decision-making: a model for clinical practice', Journal of General Internal Medicine, 27(10), pp. 1361–1367. https://doi.org/10.1007/s11606-012-2077-6.

Fontaine, S. (2018). The role of reflective practice in professional development. *Vet. Nurs. J.* 9 (7): 340–347. https://doi.org/10.12968/vetn.2018.9.7.340.

Goldberg, K. (2016). Veterinary hospice and palliative care: a comprehensive review of the literature. *Vet. Rec.* 178 (15): 369–374. https://doi.org/10.1136/vr.103459.

Hernandez, E., Fawcett, A., Brouwer, E. et al. (2018). Speaking up: veterinary ethical responsibilities and animal welfare issues in everyday practice. *Animals (Basel)* 8 (1): 15. https://doi.org/10.3390/ani8010015.

Hewson, C. (2014). Grief for pets – part 1: overview and some false assumptions. *Vet. Nurs. J.* 29 (9): 302–305. https://doi.org/10.1111/vnj.12175.

Hewson, C. (2015). Grief for pets. Part 3: supporting clients. *Vet. Nurs. J.* 30 (1): 26–30. https://doi.org/10.1080/17415349.2014.983790.

Horne, J., Weinman, J., Barber, N. and Elliott, R. (2005). *Concordance, Adherence and Compliance in Medicine Taking.* London: National Co-ordinating Centre for NHS Service Delivery and Organisation.

Institute for Healthcare Improvement (n.d.). Huddles. http://www.ihi.org/resources/Pages/Tools/Huddles.aspx (accessed 6 January 2022).

Jordan, J.L., Ellis, S.J., and Chambers, R. (2002). Defining shared decision making and concordance: are they one and the same? *Postgrad. Med. J.* 78 (921): 383–384. https://doi.org/10.1136/pmj.78.921.383.

Kerrigan, L. (2020). How to conduct an effective patient handover. *Vet. Nurs. J.* 11 (1): 4–7. https://doi.org/10.12968/vetn.2020.11.1.4.

Kerrigan, L. (2013). Veterinary palliative and hospice care – making the transition from 'cure' to 'care'. *Vet. Nurs. J.* 4 (6): 316–321. https://doi.org/10.12968/vetn.2013.4.6.316.

Kerrigan, L. (2014). In-home hospice provision – a viable option for veterinary palliative care? *Vet. Nurs. J.* 5 (3): 146–151. https://doi.org/10.12968/vetn.2014.5.3.146.

Macdonald, J., Gray, C., and Robbé, I. (2021). The development of a veterinary nurse-client communication matrix. *MedEdPublish* 10 (1): https://doi.org/10.15694/mep.2021.000144.1.

Mackenzie, J.S. and Jeggo, M. (2019). The one health approach – why is it so important? *Trop. Med. Infect. Dis.* 4 (2): 88. https://doi.org/10.3390/tropicalmed4020088.

May, S. (2017). Reflection and our professional lives. *Companion Anim.* 22 (1): 32–36. https://doi.org/10.12968/coan.2017.22.1.32.

May, S. (2020). A step change in veterinary regulation? https://www.rcvs.org.uk/news-and-views/blog/a-step-change-in-veterinary-regulation (accessed 6 January 2022).

NICE (2007). Medicines concordance FINAL scope April 2007. https://www.nice.org.uk/guidance/cg76/documents/medicines-concordance-final-scope2 (accessed 6 January 2022).

Oxtoby, C. (2017). Building a learning culture: how quality improvement can help. http://www.rcvskblog.org/building-a-learning-culture-how-quality-improvement-can-help (accessed 6 January 2022).

Oxtoby, C. (2018). Shifting from a blame culture to a learning culture. *Companion Anim.* 23 (11): 623–627. https://doi.org/10.12968/coan.2018.23.11.623.

Packer, R.M.A., O'Neill, D.G., Fletcher, F., and Farnworth, M.J. (2020). Come for the looks, stay for the personality? A mixed methods investigation of reacquisition and owner recommendation of Bulldogs, French Bulldogs and Pugs. *PLoS One* 15 (8): e0237276. https://doi.org/10.1371/journal.pone.0237276.

Paradiso, L. and Sweeney, N. (2019). Just culture. It's more than policy. *Nursing Management (Springhouse)* 50 (6): 38–43.

Radford, A.D., Stockley, P., Silverman, J. et al. (2006). Development, teaching and evaluation of a consultation structure model for use in veterinary education. *J. Vet. Med. Educ.* 33 (1): 38–44. https://doi.org/10.3138/jvme.33.1.38.

Robinson, D. (2019). The 2019 Survey of the Veterinary Nursing Profession. https://www.rcvs.org.uk/news-and-views/publications/the-2019-survey-of-the-veterinary-nursing-profession (accessed 6 January 2022).

Royal College of Surgeons of England. (2019). Be dog safe, warns surgeon as NHS figures show an increase in hospital admissions for dog bites; averaging at nearly 8000 a year. https://www.rcseng.ac.uk/news-and-events/media-centre/press-releases/be-dog-safe (accessed 6 January 2022).

Royal College of Veterinary Surgeons. (2018). Communication and consent guidance refined. https://www.rcvs.org.uk/news-and-views/news/communication-and-consent-guidance-refined (accessed 6 January 2022).

Royal College of Veterinary Surgeons. (2020a). Code of Professional Conduct for Veterinary Surgeons. Communication and consent. https://www.rcvs.org.uk/setting-standards/advice-and-guidance/code-of-professional-conduct-for-veterinary-surgeons/supporting-guidance/communication-and-consent (accessed 6 January 2022).

Royal College of Veterinary Surgeons. (2020b). RCVS Legislation Working Party Report to Council. https://www.rcvs.org.uk/document-library/rcvs-legislation-working-party-report-to-council-2020/ (accessed 31 January 2022).

Royal College of Veterinary Surgeons. (2021). Code of Professional Conduct for Veterinary Nurses: Professional responsibilities. 1. Veterinary Nurses and Animals. https://www.rcvs.org.uk/setting-standards/advice-and-guidance/code-of-professional-conduct-for-veterinary-nurses (accessed 6 January 2022).

Schwalbe, C.S., Oh, H.Y., and Zweben, A. (2014). Sustaining motivational interviewing: a meta-analysis of training studies. *Addiction* 109 (8): 1287–1294. https://doi.org/10.1111/add.12558.

The British Veterinary Association. (2019). *The vet-led team.* https://www.bva.co.uk/take-action/our-policies/the-vet-led-team (accessed 6 January 2022).

The British Veterinary Association. (2021). *Consultation response: BVA response to RCVS Legislation Working Party recommendations.* https://www.bva.co.uk/media/3980/lwp-response.pdf (accessed 6 January 2022).

The Queen's Nursing Institute (2009). *2020 Vision: Focusing on the Future of District Nursing.* https://www.qni.org.uk/resources/2020-vision-focusing-future-district-nursing (accessed 6 January 2022).

Villalobos, A. (2008). *The "HHHHHMM" Quality of Life Scale.* Pawspice. https://pawspice.com/q-of-l-care/new-page.html (accessed 6 January 2022).

VN Futures. (2016). Report and Action Plan. https://www.vnfutures.org.uk/download/vn-futures-report-and-action-plan/?wpdmdl=5043&masterkey= (accessed 6 January 2022).

Wallace, S. and May, S.A. (2016). Assessing and enhancing quality through outcomes based continuing professional development (CPD): a review of current practice. *Vet. Rec.* 179 (20): 515–520. https://doi.org/10.1136/vr.103862.

Further Reading

Adams, V. (2019). Developing your role in hospice and palliative care. Today's Veterinary Nurse. https://todaysveterinarynurse.com/articles/career-challenges-developing-your-role-in-hospice-and-palliative-care (accessed 6 January 2022).

Advocacy Focus (n.d.). What is advocacy? https://www.advocacyfocus.org.uk/understanding-advocacy (accessed 6 January 2022).

American Animal Hospital Association (n.d.). Animal versus human hospice care. https://www.aaha.org/aaha-guidelines/end-of-life-care/animal-versus-human-hospice-care (accessed 6 January 2022).

Boysen, P.G., 2nd(2013). Just culture: a foundation for balanced accountability and patient safety. *Ochsner J.* 13 (3): 400–406.

Chapman, H. (2018). Nursing theories 4: adherence and concordance. *Nurs. Times* 114 (2): 50.

Coulter, A. (1999). Paternalism or partnership? Patients have grown up – and there's no going back. *Br. Med. J. (Clin. Res. Ed.)* 319 (7212): 719–720. https://doi.org/10.1136/bmj.319.7212.719.

Fraser, M. (2019). An overview of decision-making in veterinary nursing. *Vet. Nurs. J.* 10 (9): https://doi.org/10.12968/vetn.2019.10.9.460.

Gray, C.A. (2020). Informed consent – more than a signature? Improving the consent process in practice. *Vet. Nurs. J.* 35 (4): 93–95. http://doi.org/10.1080/17415349.2020.1730284.

Hewson, C. (2014). Grief for pets – part 2: avoiding compassion fatigue. *Vet. Nurs. J.* 29 (12): 388–391. https://doi.org/10.1111/vnj.12199.

Hewson, C. (2015). End-of-life care: the why and how of animal hospice. *Vet. Nurs. J.* 30 (10): 287–289. https://doi.org/10.1080/17415349.2015.1082452.

Kerrigan, L. (2020). Creating a just and learning culture through staff support. *Vet. Nurs. J.* 11 (2): 52–55. https://doi.org/10.12968/vetn.2020.11.2.52.

Kitchen, S. (1999). An appraisal of methods of reflection and clinical supervision. *Br. J. Theatr. Nurs.* 9 (7): 313–317. https://doi.org/10.1177/175045899900900704.

Macdonald, J. (2015). Your wellbeing (and mind) matters to us! *Vet. Nurs. J.* 30 (12): 343–344. https://doi.org/10.1080/17415349.2015.1099490.

Macdonald, J. (2019). Emerging role of community nursing. *Feline Focus.* 5 (11): 301–306.

Macdonald, J. and Gray, C. (2014). 'Informed consent' – how do we get it right? *Vet. Nurs. J.* 29 (3): 101–103. http://doi.org/10.1111/vnj.12123.

NHS Resolution (2019). Being Fair Report. https://resolution.nhs.uk/resources/being-fair-report (accessed 6 January 2022).

NHS Resolution (2019). Being Fair leaflet. https://resolution.nhs.uk/wp-content/uploads/2019/07/NHS-Resolution_Being-fair-Website2.pdf (accessed 6 January 2022).

Oxtoby, C., Ferguson, E., White, K., and Mossop, L. (2015). We need to talk about error: causes and types of error in veterinary practice. *Vet. Rec.* 177: https://doi.org/10.1136/vr.103331.

Rollnick, S., Miller, W., and Butler, C. (2008). *Motivational Interviewing in Healthcare. Helping Patients Change Behavior*. New York: Guildford Press.

Royal College of Nursing. (2019). How motivational interviewing works. https://www.rcn.org.uk/clinical-topics/supporting-behaviour-change/motivational-interviewing (accessed 6 January 2022).

Royal College of Veterinary Surgeons. (2017). Gauging the extent of 'blame culture' within the veterinary professions. https://www.rcvs.org.uk/news-and-views/news/gauging-the-extent-of-blame-culture (accessed 6 January 2022).

Royal Pharmaceutical Society of Great Britain (1997). *From Compliance to Concordance. Achieving Shared Goals in Medicine Taking*. London: RPSGB.

Smith, N. (2016). A questionnaire based study to assess compassion fatigue in UK practising veterinary nurses. *Vet. Nurs. J.* 7 (7): https://doi.org/10.12968/vetn.2016.7.7.418.

The Blue Cross (n.d.). *Pet bereavement and pet loss*. https://www.bluecross.org.uk/pet-bereavement-and-pet-loss (accessed 6 January 2022).

Thompson-Hughes, J. (2019). Burnout and compassion fatigue within veterinary nursing: a literature review. *Vet. Nurs. J.* 34 (10): 266–268. https://doi.org/10.1080/17415349.2019.1646620.

WHO. (2020). Palliative care. https://www.who.int/health-topics/palliative-care.

6 The Veterinary Nurse Educator

Hilary Orpet and Andrea Jeffery

This chapter begins by considering what it is that veterinary nurses need to know in order for them to develop a unique body of knowledge in their role. It continues by reviewing how learners learn and the importance that the alignment of teaching and learning has in this. This includes the exploration of learning outcomes, teaching activities and the importance of assessment for achievement. The chapter then moves on to consider the importance of experiential learning and the stages of learning as veterinary nurses move through their careers from student through to expert practitioners, and how the development of critical thinking skills can support learning. The final stages of the chapter review how we can support students in the clinical environment and the important role that a preceptor plays as students become registered veterinary nurses (RVNs) and the development of their careers.

What do Veterinary Nurses Need to Know?

A unique body of knowledge is one of the criteria that defines a profession (Clarke 2012). In veterinary nursing, this 'unique body of knowledge' such as anatomy and physiology, pharmacology, medical diseases, and surgical conditions is shared with other veterinary and medical professionals. It is therefore important to identify the aspects of this body of knowledge that are unique to veterinary nursing. Veterinary nurses are often defined by the technical skills they can perform under Schedule 3 of the Veterinary Surgeons Act (1966) (Figure 6.1), but this is such a small area of the veterinary nurse's role.

Providing evidence-based patient care consumes the majority of the veterinary nurse's time in addition to supporting the owners of the animal, and providing expert advice concerning the general husbandry and care of the animal. Carrying out a nursing patient assessment to identify the needs and requirements of the patient and then creating a plan of care to achieve those goals, as well as understanding the normal routine of the animal in order to provide individual care, play a much bigger part in the role of the veterinary nurse. Entering the register of

Professionalism and Reflection in Veterinary Nursing, First Edition.
Edited by Sue Badger and Andrea Jeffery.
© 2022 John Wiley & Sons Ltd. Published 2022 by John Wiley & Sons Ltd.
Companion website: www.wiley.com/go/badger/professionalism-veterinary-nursing

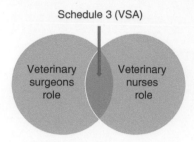

Figure 6.1   Veterinary nurses are often defined by Schedule 3 (Veterinary Surgeons Act 1966) activities.

veterinary nurses held by the Royal College of Veterinary Surgeons (RCVS) should not be the end point of our studies. It is our professional duty to continue to update and maintain our clinical and professional knowledge. Instilling this idea of life-long learning into the current generation of students is essential for the development of the profession. This needs to start at the initial stages of training to become a veterinary nurse.

How do Learners Learn?

Understanding how learners learn is perhaps an important place to start when considering how we teach or perhaps how we 'facilitate learning'. Learning styles that were once popular often grouped students into specific categories: visual, auditory, or kinaesthetic, and later 'reading and writing' learners (Petty 2010) or perhaps reflective, active, pragmatic, or theorist learner types (Honey and Mumford 1995). You could take a short test and be told you are a reflective learner or perhaps an auditory learner, categorising you into one style. While we may have a tendency towards one style or another, we probably use a variety of styles depending on the activity involved (Biggs and Tang 2011). The teaching approach to accommodate these different styles is to use a variety of activities that would appeal to each style of learning. This can become impracticable when trying to cover the required content. Instead we should be considering designing various activities that relate to the content. For example, you do not teach someone to handle and restrain a dog for an injection in the classroom via a lecture. You show them and allow them to practise on toy in a practical session. Do not give a lecture on the classification of disinfectants; instead, provide them with the resources to create a chart, perhaps working together in a group to get the task done. In this way we can move away from teacher-focused 'passive' learning to student-focused 'active' learning. The role the educators now play should be in facilitating the learning rather than teaching.

Teaching or Facilitating Learning?

Traditionally teaching has been very teacher-focused, with lecturers preparing sessions involving them telling the students what they know (Long and Lock 2010).

While this passive style of learning is very popular with students, it is often difficult to gauge the level of engagement let alone the learning that may take place. This method is also easy for the teacher – they just need to tell the students everything they know about a particular topic. The traditional method of learning by attending lectures is often perceived by students to be effective learning, particularly if the lecturer has an engaging style of delivery (Carpenter et al. 2020).

The interesting aspect is that teachers may deliver sessions in slightly different ways – if you have ever had to deliver someone else's lecture you will have recognised this. Teachers teach differently in the same way that students learn differently. If we deliver the information via one-way communication, we hope that students will be engaged, and some students will say they learn best by listening to somebody. We then assess them and use this as a test of whether the students have learned information from our lectures, when in actual fact most students will cram this information last minute just before the assessment. So what was the use of our lectures apart from giving them information which they could quite easily read themselves?

The way the student *approaches* learning plays an important part in how effective they are in learning. A surface approach often means the student is relying on rote learning and last-minute 'cramming' to be able to be successful in the end assessment. A deep approach to learning is more effective as the student understands the key concepts and can then apply these to different scenarios. Our patients may present with similar conditions but the individual care they require may be very different. How we design our teaching is important, we need to include activities that encourage deep learning, and this is the foundation of problem-based learning that many medical schools use (Albanese 2010). If we choose to deliver the content as a series of lectures, the surface learner will often take the easy route, passively sitting in a lecture, occasionally underlining or highlighting key words. At assessment time the surface learner student tries to memorise the content of the lecture to regurgitate in the examination. The deep learner in the lecture may also be highlighting text, but also writing questions which later help them to construct meaning and underlying themes from the material delivered. That same student may revisit the topic over the next few days and weeks to ensure they have a good understanding of the material. When it come to the assessment, they can usually expand further on their answers, demonstrating how well they know the topic. The surface learner may have been able to provide information relevant to the topic but will fail to provide depth to their answer. Fortunately, the deep approach works well for application of knowledge type questions as well as recall, such as multiple-choice questions.

Active learning has become more popular in recent years, with flipped classrooms (Erbil 2020), peer-to-peer interactions, and allowing the student to formatively complete activities related to the learning outcomes as a practise for the summative assessment. We need to consider what is it that the students need to learn, and design activities that enable the students to actively engage with the information via problem-solving or discussion. We then need to assess them in an appropriate way in order to measure the achievement of intended outcomes and be satisfied that they have reached the required standard.

Aligning Our Teaching and Learning

This connection between the programme aims and objectives, the intended learning outcomes, the teaching and learning activities, and the final assessment is called constructive alignment (Biggs and Tang 2011). The 'constructive' part refers to the meaning the students should gain from engaging in the learning activities (Figure 6.2).

When we design the teaching activities, we need to consider what the intended outcome is. What assessment do we create that will allow us to make the judgement on their performance to meet the outcome? What activities can we design so that the student can practise before they are assessed? What are the intended learning outcomes that will guide the student to complete these activities? So rather than starting with the learning outcomes:

intended learning outcomes > learning activities > assessment > outcome

we flip this and start at the end point:

outcome > assessment > learning activities > intended learning outcomes

The assessment should then be able to measure the learning outcomes and this ensures the activities are designed so that the student can attain the learning outcome by undertaking appropriate assessment. This is known as outcomes-based assessment. Using the example of disinfection and sterilisation, the student may be required to produce a report detailing the evidence base on the use of different methods of disinfection and sterilisation as a learning activity and then produce a recommended plan of how this can effectively be carried out in the practice as the summative assessment.

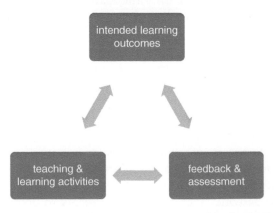

Figure 6.2   Constructive alignment. Source: Adapted from Biggs and Tang (2011).

Learning Outcomes

If you want a student to 'understand the principles of disinfection and sterilisation', how will you measure this? You can assess them, but depending on the type of assessment you may just get 'recall' rather than 'understand'. Consider what you want a veterinary nurse to be able to do once qualified? What type of assessment will enable you to make the judgement on whether the veterinary nurse can complete the skill or competency with the required level of underpinning knowledge? Why do you want the veterinary nurse to 'understand the principles of disinfection and sterilisation'? A veterinary nurse must have the important underpinning knowledge to carry out successful cleaning, disinfection and sterilisation in the practice. So perhaps 'utilising the principles of disinfection and sterilisation, create a practice infection control protocol'. This learning outcome describes the activity (utilise) the object (principles of disinfection and sterilisation) and then puts it into context (infection control in the practice) (Biggs and Tang 2011).

Module learning outcomes are much broader and will cover a wider range of activities, but the lesson learning outcomes can be more specific. If these are well written, you can turn them into questions – then there is no doubt that what is in the examination was covered in the module!

Writing good learning outcomes ensure that it is clear what the students need to learn and to what cognitive level (declarative knowledge) but also what they need to be able to do with the knowledge (functional knowledge) (Biggs and Tang 2011). They are statements that describe the knowledge or skills that the students should acquire by the end of a learning session. Bloom's taxonomy has frequently been used been used to create learning outcomes in education (Bloom et al. 1956). Anderson and Krathwohl's revision of Bloom's taxonomy in 2001 moved to changing the nouns to verbs (see Table 6.1) (Krathwohl 2002). The revised edition suggests that evaluation should come prior to creation or synthesis.

There is an expectation that as the student progresses to the higher levels of the course, the learning outcomes also increase in cognitive complexity. While the lower levels of Bloom's taxonomy indicate an accumulation of knowledge, in addition there is an expectation that in the higher levels of the course the learning outcomes should indicate the application of the knowledge gained (Bates 2016).

Table 6.1   Anderson and Krathwohl's revision of Bloom's taxonomy.

Bloom's taxonomy 1956	Anderson and Krathwohl's revision of Bloom's 2001
Knowledge	Remember
Comprehension	Understand
Application	Apply
Analysis	Analyse
Synthesis	Evaluate
Evaluation	Create

Source: Adapted from Armstrong (2010).

Often in veterinary nursing courses, topics are introduced at all stages of the course, rather than introduced at the start and then built on from the first year. The verbs used in the writing of the learning outcomes should then be appropriate to the existing knowledge the student has on a topic. For example, sterilisation is often taught within theatre practice and usually not in the first year, so the learner will first need to 'list' the different types of sterilisation before they can 'apply' their knowledge to a scenario.

Veterinary nursing and veterinary medicine are a competency-driven style of education. The RCVS day one skills (RCVS 2016 and competencies (RCVS 2014) provide the requirements to enter the register for both veterinary surgeons and veterinary nurses. However, if we just limit the learning outcomes to competencies and skills, we are limiting the cognitive level required for further and higher education. We must also take into account the academic level at which the students are working. The Framework for Higher Education Qualifications (FHEQ) descriptors indicates the level of the final qualification (Quality Assurance Agency 2014). In higher education, students typically start at level 4 during their first year and progress to level 5 for Foundation degrees and level 6 for BSc degrees. These levels set the expected standards that students should be working at, irrespective of the degree course they are on. Similarly, in further education the Regulated Qualification Framework (Ofqual 2017) identifies the descriptors for the different levels, with the veterinary nursing diploma mostly at level 3.

Teaching Activities

Problem-based learning (PBL) is popular in medical schools, with the entire curriculum being delivered as PBL (Wood 2003). Scenarios or case presentations are used to provide context for the students to acquire knowledge about the basic sciences (Albanese 2010). Teamwork is key and students take on different roles within the group to facilitate learning. An example of this in veterinary nursing could be a cat that is admitted after a road traffic accident with a fractured pelvis. The topics explored in this one scenario might be: water distribution in the body and effects of shock, bone composition and healing, drugs used for analgesia, and maybe anaesthesia, and their effects and probably many others. The scenario provides the context and reason for learning the required knowledge.

Flipped classrooms are where the students are provided with material to read or a short video to watch providing the background information (Erbil 2020; Halasa et al. 2020). Class time is then spent in active learning through discussion and clarification. Students may be required to produce material in small groups such as the completion of charts or tables.

Peer learning is particularly useful to get students working together on a common goal. Team-based learning is another active learning method whereby the group first completes preparatory activities individually before the session. Then, in the session they complete an individual multiple-choice test and group multiple-choice tests to hold them accountable for their preparation in stage one. This part of the session enables peer teaching to ensure all the group are up to speed. The third stage then involves application of their knowledge to a problem (Parmalee and Michaelsen 2010).

Peer assessment is an important professional skill for veterinary nurses in learning to provide constructive feedback. These skills are essential within the clinics especially when managing a team.

Assessment for Achievement

Assessment is often the endpoint of learning and it has been suggested that 'assessment drives learning' (Wood 2009; Wormald et al. 2009). Students are driven to learn to the exam rather than focus on understanding the material and utilising a deeper level of learning to be able to apply their knowledge in the clinical environment. A good assessment will not encourage rote learning but rather extract how well the student can apply their knowledge. While there are always going to be areas that require Bloom's lower cognitive level of 'remember', in practice, the skills of deduction, problem-solving, and clinical reasoning are essential for good patient care. Whilst you will have learnt a list of nursing interventions for looking after a cat with a fractured pelvis, you still need to make a judgement on which of those activities are going to be appropriate for the individual patient in your care.

Designing the assessment for a competency-based programme is easy if the learning outcomes are written well. For example, 'Identify the muscles commonly used for intramuscular injection.' In written format, the assessment could be a diagram that requires labelling. In a practical assessment this could be part of a scenario that might include calculating the dose required and injecting into the correct muscle in the hind limb. It is essential that the learning outcomes align with the assessment activities. In this way, the students can use the learning outcomes from which to revise.

Formative and Summative Assessment

Formative assessment is essential for helping students to be able to practise the assessment and obtain feedback. This has more recently been termed 'feedforward' as it is intended to commend areas which are well done and also suggest areas for improvement going forward. Students can learn from the 'feedback' and improve for the summative assessment activities. There are usually no consequences if the student is failing to meet the required standard in formative assessment, but it does enable constructive feedback to be provided to the student. Also, having the opportunity to practise in a low-stakes environment reduces stress levels.

Summative assessment is required for the purposes of making a judgement on the ability of the students to progress or for certification purposes. While feedback is routinely provided for summative assessment it can often indicate the justification of the mark rather than developing the student. It may be that this type of assessment may not be encountered again, such as in finals, but if the students are likely to have to re-sit the component, they need to know where they went wrong.

Blueprinting and Mapping

The assessment should address the broad learning outcomes and ensure a wide range of topics are covered. Every examination should have a blueprint indicating the topics or objectives covered and the cognitive domain level addressed by the assessment. For example, a module on surgical nursing might include some multiple choice questions (MCQs) which cover recall, but you might want to incorporate some higher-level activities utilising problem-solving questions or application of knowledge to a nursing scenario. An Objective Structured Clinical Examination (OSCE) should be mapped to the skills and competencies required by the professional body such as the RCVS. In veterinary nursing we have a clearly structured format of ensuring students gain the skills they require by way of the RCVS Nursing Progress Log or similar electronic records of competency. The OSCE should therefore then sample the range of skills acquired to ensure the students have reached the required standard.

Benefits and Challenges of Assessment Types

Reliability and validity are often referred to regarding forms of assessment. A reliable assessment will be able to provide consistent scores when used with different groups of learners. A highly reliable assessment will often have a coefficient score of 0.80 where 0 = no reliability to 1 = perfect reliability. The reliability increases with longer examinations, for example an OSCE lasting one hour has a coefficient of 0.54 while an OSCE of four hours has a coefficient of 0.82 (van der Vleuten and Schuwirth 2005). These results were from a single study but provides comparative data to enable decision-making on length of testing time. Obviously a longer OSCE will enable increased sampling of the skills and therefore be more predictive of the reliability of the examination in making a judgement on the student's practical skills.

The validity of the assessment refers to whether the assessment actually measures what it is supposed to (van der Vleuten and Schuwirth 2005). If you want to measure the clinical ability of a student, then a practical examination is going to be more valid than a written examination.

Multiple Choice Questions (MCQs)

MCQs are a good way of assessing a wide range of the content. A variety of software programmes can be used to mark paper-based answer sheets and online tests can be set up easily in a range of different platforms. The ideal MCQ should be single best answer (Sam et al. 2016) where the distractors could be possible but are not the best answer available. This type of question is much better at discriminating than easily eliminated distractors. Good students have often said the distractors can confuse them and they utilise the cover-up method – hiding the distractors and trying to answer the question alone.

Extended Matching Questions (EMQs)

Extended Matching Questions are often used in medical education to explore the students' knowledge about a range of conditions. The topic theme is given, e.g. wound care in dogs. Then a list of potential answers are provided (minimum of 8). For this example, it may be a list of dressings. The questions are then a number (around 5) of scenarios or vignettes which are then provided and the student is required to select from the 8 possible answers. While these can assess greater depth and application than an MCQ as more than one answer can be correct, they are more labour-intensive to create and it is not easy to cover all areas of the curriculum. An advantage is that they can be marked electronically in the same way as MCQs.

Short Answer Questions – Problem-Solving or Recall

Many people used short answer questions for recall. 'List the 12 cranial nerves', 'Identify 5 muscles that may be injected into'. Scenario-based questions are useful to assess more depth of knowledge and how well they can apply what they know. The question may have a number of sub-sections (a, b, c, etc.) which if written well can guide the student to a deeper level of understanding. A good model answer is important and recognition that the student may present plausible answers not considered in the model answer. This also means the exams cannot be electronically marked although there are software systems that use a type of data mining to evaluate the answers (Süzen et al. 2020).

Presentations – Slides/Posters

Oral presentations are useful to assess both communication and knowledge of a topic. The student can be asked to present their ideas using Powerpoint™ slides. The presentation can be by an individual or by a small group. The marking scheme should take into account everyone's input into the task and peer review can be also integrated. Poster presentations are useful to ensure conciseness and focus on the topic. Research projects are often presented in this way, allowing the student to communicate the key aspects of their project. This method of presenting research is now common at conferences and utilising it as part of the assessment helps to prepare the students for lifelong learning. Marking is more achievable and can be completed on the day using specific rubrics assessing content, presentation, and also the student's ability to answer questions on their project.

Assignments

Assignments in the form of essays or reports are commonplace in most courses. They allow greater depth of knowledge to be explored and test the student's ability to communicate in a coherent and logical manner. Patient care reports are useful, and students can be encouraged to publish if the report is well written.

Practical Assessment – OSCEs, DOPS, mini-CEX

Assessment of practical skills in veterinary medicine is key in confirming competency. Assessment in the workplace introduces high validity as the tasks are performed in the clinical environment often involving live patients. Unfortunately, the unpredictability of assessment opportunities and the variation in patients lowers the reliability of the assessment.

OSCEs are practical assessments, which are standardised ensuring that every student completes the same scenario and same task. There are typically 10–20 stations, each lasting around 5–6 minutes. The marking is completed using checklists with a global rating scale to indicate overall performance. There is high reliability if enough tasks are sampled and examiners must be trained to ensure consistency. The resources and staffing are costly but it is a fair method to assess a number of students. While the scenarios and tasks are meant to represent the activities in the workplace, it is not normal to undertake a series of tasks in a limited 5-minute time frame.

Direct Observation of Procedural Skills (DOPS) are practical assessments in the workplace. The student is assessed by a generic form that considers key aspects of performing the task such as health and safety, animal welfare, technical ability and communication. The student is graded as competent or not yet competent and may be given a number of opportunities to be reassessed.

Mini-clinical examinations (mini-CEX) are similar to DOPS but involve a live patient rather than just performing a task. In medical education these are often used to assess how the student interacts with a patient, and how they take a clinical history and perform a clinical examination.

The Clinical Classroom

The knowledge base for veterinary nurses is wide-ranging, with anatomy and physiology providing a base to build upon aspects of nursing care and diagnostic procedures. This is not learnt in isolation in classroom but combined with the experiences of placement activities to provide a more enriched learning experience (Morris and Blaney 2010). Experiential learning is core to veterinary nursing. Being able to apply the knowledge learnt in the classroom to the nursing care provided and similarly, taking those experiences of working in the practice back to the classroom, helps to make sense of the concepts and knowledge encountered. Another effect of undertaking practical placements is that veterinary nurses have a good idea of what they need to know to be successful in the clinic rather than learning topics in isolation in a classroom for three years.

Transformational learning is making sense of experiences by utilising disorientating dilemmas to challenge student's thinking (Bates 2016). The comparatively large amount of practical placement required by the regulatory body lends itself to utilising this educational theory in veterinary nursing. Ensuring that students take time to understand the meaning of the experiences they have in practice helps to develop the autonomous thinker (Mezirow 1997).

Mezirow Model (Figure 6.3)

- *Experience of life* – we need to consider what previous experiences, knowledge, and skills our learners enter veterinary nursing education with. In any educational setting we should always try to gauge the level of our leaners to ensure what we deliver is appropriate to their needs.
- *Critical reflection* – this is an essential aspect of adult learning, questioning what we see and do. So much of veterinary education is taught in a passive way and the students are encouraged to learn a lot of material. When do we allow the students to question what we are teaching them? We should ensure we provide those 'stop and think' sessions to allow students to reflect on the concepts covered.
- *Rational discourse* – encourages the discussion between teachers and students to explore the learner's beliefs and values in relation to the content being delivered. Provide opportunities for students to discuss what they have seen in the practice and this will enable them to have a better understanding. Encouraging these critical thinking skills will enhance their learning.

It is important to ensure that the experiences the student has in the clinical placement are incorporated into the classroom activities. This can be achieved by encouraging students to relate the knowledge being learnt in the classroom to

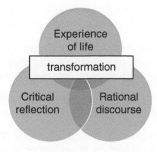

Figure 6.3   Mezirow model.

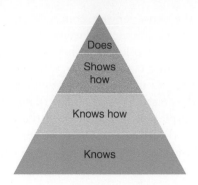

Figure 6.4   Miller's pyramid. Source: Adapted from Miller (1990).

patients they have seen. This model works well for an apprenticeship style or vocational training. True meaning and understanding can be then taken further if the student undertakes further analysis of the experience, challenging the methods used, and relating to an evidence base to improve patient care.

The other aspect to consider is how do we know when someone is competent? Miller's pyramid is often referred to as a model for assessing clinical competence (Miller 1990) (Figure 6.4). The underpinning knowledge required is at the bottom level (knows). Above this is the level of initial competence (knows how) and then the level of performance (shows how) and finally the top level, indicating the normal routine performance of the qualified practitioner.

Benner developed a competency scale for student nurses in human-centred nursing based on Dreyfus's model of skill acquisition (Benner 1984; Dreyfus 2004). She indicated that the new graduate nurse would be at the level of advanced beginner and that with one to two years' experience would then reach the level of competence.

The descriptors of competency help the assessor to make a judgement on the performance of the nurse.

Stage of Competence	Description
Novice	Has little experience and relies on rules to help perform tasks, e.g. 'Tell me what I need to do and I'll do it.'
Advanced beginner	Demonstrates acceptable performance based on prior experiences and able to recognise recurring meaningful components.
Competent	Experience in the day-to-day situations. Gains perspective from planning own actions based on conscious and analytical thinking. More aware of long-term goals and helps to achieve greater efficiency and organisation.
Proficient	Perceives and understands situations as whole part. Learns from previous experiences what to expect in certain situations and how to modify plans.
Expert	Has an intuitive grasp of clinical situations. Performance of task is fluid, flexible, and highly proficient. No longer relies on guidelines to connect situations and determine actions.

Developing Critical Thinking Skills

When we use the term 'critical thinking' with regard to students and how we wish them to think, it is important that we are clear in the definition ourselves and that we use it appropriately. This ensures that what we wish to develop in our students is actually critical thinking. Other interrelated concepts are clinical judgement and clinical reasoning. All three are concepts for student (SVNs) and registered veterinary nurses (RVNs) to be familiar with as they undertake evidence-based veterinary nursing practice. Differentiating between and understanding these concepts is important before trying to apply them within clinical practice.

Definitions

Critical thinking is a process of thinking based on evidence and science and not on guesswork or assumptions and it is not a discipline-specific term. There is wide-ranging literature about it and published tools that can be used to assess it (Victor-Chmil 2013). Clinical reasoning is the use of critical thinking in a clinical setting or when considering a clinical patient in a teaching or learning environment. Clinical reasoning skills will differ depending on the level of knowledge and experience of those undertaking it, but regardless of this it is always based on evidence.

The reason that it is important to develop critical thinking and clinical reasoning skills as a student or an RVN is that they are needed in order to make a sound clinical nursing judgement regarding their patients. According to Tanner (2006), whose primary research was the application of clinical judgement from a nursing perspective, there are five assumptions of clinical judgement within nursing, which have been translated here to reflect the veterinary patient and the client:

- Clinical judgement is influenced by the nurse experience as well as the objective data.
- Clinical judgement includes the nurse's knowledge about the patient and how they respond, as well as engaging with the client and understanding their concerns.
- Clinical judgement is influenced by the context and the environment in which the nursing is taking place.
- When making a clinical judgement nurses use a variety of reasoning patterns (depending on experience and situation).
- Clinical judgement improves through review, reflection, learning, and application.

The five assumptions of nursing clinical judgement have a holistic approach to clinical judgement and take into account the patient, client, the nurse and the nursing team as well as other members of the veterinary team. The nurse, when making a clinical judgement, is going through a process of noticing, interpreting, responding, and reflecting (Victor-Chmil 2013, p. 35).

Application

It is important that critical thinking, clinical reasoning, and clinical judgement skills (3Cs) are embedded into the curriculum from the start of a programme of study, be that in further or higher education. The skills can be implicitly and explicitly embedded throughout each year of study (DeSimone 2006). The process and the skills needed for it to happen then become an integral part of the approach to nursing, regardless of the situation.

If we consider the type of learning and the curriculum content within a veterinary nursing programme of study and where the 3Cs could be embedded:

- as an introduction to professional nursing practice (at the start of programme and ongoing throughout all years)
- when teaching clinical nursing skills (all years)
- when considering a patient with a known medical or surgical condition and what the nursing care interventions might be (this could be basic nursing care at the start of learning through to complex patient needs later in a curriculum)
- when using care plans to determine the similarities and differences of two patients with similar conditions and the clients of those patients (all years)
- as part of a written analysis of a nursing issue (all years)
- in research skills and projects
- when teaching about analysis of an ethical nursing dilemma.

These are some examples, but it is important that a culture of 3Cs runs vertically and horizontally through any curriculum or programme of professional development. Providing the tools to seek the best evidence is the basis for this to happen.

DeSimone (2006) embedded the 3Cs within a nursing leadership and management module, where there was the need for a written analysis of the design, implementation, and evaluation of a 'change' project with the intention of change implementation. Managing change within a veterinary environment is an important leadership and management skill and is an area where more nurses are becoming involved, particularly around the review of significant events and near misses (Oxtoby and Mossop 2019). The introduction of the Veterinary Defence Society (VDS) Vetsafe reporting system has helped facilitate this type of review and the veterinary nurse's role is vital in this process.

Emotional Intelligence and Critical Thinking

Emotional intelligence is the understanding and management of emotional thoughts in ourselves and others (Mayer et al. 2008; Akerjordet and Severinsson 2010). The need to develop emotional intelligence along with critical thinking skills for nurses to deliver best patient (and client) care as part of the clinical team is important. For a nurse to be a critical thinker there also needs to be a cognitive, emotional, and professional ability. Critical thinking and emotional intelligence are clearly linked, as critical thinking is vital to the quality of an individual's emotional intelligence and both are key to the success of the professional practice of nurses (Christianson 2020).

It is important in order to develop critical thinking skills that the methods used to deliver our teaching are reviewed to ensure that this skill is developed, and if the delivery of teaching is predominantly lecture based, this opportunity may be being missed. The work undertaken by Fernandez et al. (2012) found that when emotional intelligence and critical thinking skills were integrated into an outcomes-focused curriculum, which also included student-directed learning, they were predictors of academic performance. Another approach used to promote critical thinking described by Zhang and Chen (2020) is co-operative learning. Co-operative learning is where students work together using discussion to interpret, analyse, and evaluate an area of nursing that they are studying. Co-operative learning has five basic elements;

Positive interdependence	Having a co-operative group with a common goal to complete a learning task
Individual accountability	Each learner is responsible for the success of the group as a whole
Promotive interactions	The group works together to improve teamwork
Social skills training	Through communication and negotiation with team members
Group processing	Learning from each other and reflecting on their own and the groups learning experiences

An example of co-operative learning is where students work together to divide the tasks and then present the findings together, this could apply to any aspect of a veterinary nursing curriculum where a problem-solving approach is needed. Students promote each other's contribution to the work as well as their own and hold themselves and each other accountable for their share of the work. This is not intended to create a culture of blame but one of equal accountability and ownership around the teamwork exercise being undertaken.

If a co-operative learning environment is established in the educational setting it helps students become less reliant on the 'teacher' as the only authority and start to recognise their peers as reliable sources of knowledge too. This helps build confidence in their peers and therefore, as they move into a clinical workplace, they also develop confidence in their professional peers (Austria et al. 2013). Co-operative learning can be and is applied in a clinical practical environment within veterinary nursing, perhaps more so than in a classroom setting currently. Its continued use within all learning environments will increase the skill set of the individuals and the teams within which they work (Souers et al. 2007).

An example of where co-operative learning could be used in veterinary nursing is when teaching students about anaesthesia breathing systems and how, by understanding the principles of the functions of the breathing systems, one student can explain the principle as others work collaboratively to assemble the system using this principles-based approach.

Supporting the Student in the Clinical Environment

Unconscious (Implicit) Bias in Veterinary Nursing

The understanding of what unconscious (implicit) bias is and why it is important for veterinary nurses to be aware of will raise awareness of something, which as individual practitioners we may not have been educated in or are oblivious to. It can influence our behaviour towards our team members, clients, and potentially our patients. Unconscious bias has been found to impact the interpersonal relationships that human-centred nurses have with their clients (Gatewood et al. 2019). It is important during student nurse education that unconscious bias is considered as part of the curriculum. Understanding that it exists and how it might impact upon communication with others is an important part of developing as a professional practitioner.

Harvard University hosts a 'not for profit' initiative called the Implicit Association Test (IAT) as a method of assessing unconscious bias across a wide range of topics including testing for bias against age, weight, sexuality, race, gender, and skin tone. The IAT is an online test, which measures the speed of the reaction time of an individual to react to images and words on the screen to determine bias. An example is the race IAT, where, for example, if an individual has a bias towards white people they would rapidly pair white faces on the test with positive words such as 'good' or 'success'. The IAT can be accessed via http://implicit.harvard.edu/implicit. The first step required to address any implicit bias is to recognise that it exists and taking the IAT is a simple way of determining this and then considering that if bias is present, how this can be addressed. Shultz and Baker (2017) introduced an unconscious bias training activity with a group of human-centred nurses helping them to recognise that it exists and develop strategies to manage their own personal biases in their professional roles.

Gatewood et al. (2019) describe implementing a learning activity around implicit bias in four human-centred nursing colleges across the USA. The overall number of participants was 110 and the learning objective set was to summarise the effect that implicit bias has on quality of care. Each individual undertook the IAT to determine if they had any biases. They were then asked to consider how these biases may have influenced or could, in the future, influence their approach to nursing care. In human-centred nursing, the care is obviously delivered to other humans, but this exercise is of value in veterinary nursing in terms of the client interactions nurses have, particularly around obtaining information regarding their pets when they are being hospitalised, but more importantly, when determining a successful home care plan for the patient when they are discharged back into the care of the client.

The structure and process of the learning activity undertaken by the nursing students (n = 110) in the Gatewood et al. study was a three-step process:

Step one – preparation for the students	Watch a video to learn about implicit bias and the IAT Read an article regarding implicit bias in health care
Step two – complete IAT	Complete one IAT test from the list provided by the authors
Step three – discussion activity	Students share which IAT they did (not what their bias was) and say what they learnt about themselves from the IAT Did the result surprise the student – why/why not? Students to say what actions they can take as individuals to mitigate against their biases.

(based on Gatewood et al., 2019)

The students were not expected to disclose the IAT results in terms of their own biases. The activity started with a reminder of the 'rules of engagement' around co-operative learning before undertaking the activity. The findings of the study were that introducing the learning activity in the first year of a programme of study before the students went into clinical placement, increased the awareness of implicit bias before the students faced their patients. From a veterinary nursing perspective this not only applies to how we interact with our clients but, as mentioned at the start of this section, we also need to consider our implicit biases in relation to the veterinary teams we will be working with, as well as the students within the cohorts that we educate.

Gender Bias

The veterinary nurse workforce in the UK lacks diversity in gender, the RCVS Survey of the Veterinary Nursing Profession of 2019 had a 28.8% response rate (n = 4993) and of those 96.8% were female and 2.7% male (RCVS 2019). It is therefore important to consider the experience of male students and RVNs within both educational and clinical settings, taking into account the challenges they may face including stereotyping by others, including lecturers, peers, others in the veterinary team and clients. Work by Powers et al. (2018) in the field of human-centred nursing found that being visibly different may bring about a sense of isolation. An example cited was in relation to the teaching of the male and female reproductive systems, where there was less emphasis on the female reproductive system than the male as there was an assumption that this would be known about in more detail by the cohort. Another example of gender bias reported was regarding males being treated more critically than their female peers in terms of competence. The role of the males in the clinical setting was also a challenge, with males reporting that they were taken from one clinical task to 'help' in another area because they were stronger and could therefore help with heavier patients. The males in the study also reported clients assuming they were doctors because they were male and nursing is a female career.

The lack of gender diversity in veterinary nursing emphasises the importance of male role models and the opportunity to be able to share experiences with someone of the same gender. For those females working with other genders, avoid asking for a view from a 'male' perspective. Ensure that conversations and information sharing are gender-neutral, ensure that all students or team members are provided with the same opportunities regardless of gender (or any other bias), and where possible provide gender-specific peer support and increase access to diverse role models.

Preceptorship – What Is it and Why Is it Important?

Preceptorship is the provision of clinical orientation, support, education, and guidance which takes place at any point where there is a career transition (Ward and McComb 2017). The focus may be on the transition from student to registered professional, or when a registered professional moves from one role into another, in the same environment or a different one. The RCVS at the time of publication does not have a set of 'year one' competencies and skills which they expect new (0–12 month) RVNs to complete. This is different from veterinary science where newly qualified veterinary surgeons, as part of their professional development phase (PDP) are required to complete a set of year one competencies and skills.

While there remains a lack of parity across both professional groups as they join the veterinary team, it is important that newly qualified RVNs have support as they integrate into their new roles. Within human-centred nursing in the UK there is a well-established, formalised, and structured preceptorship programme. The aim of this section of the chapter is to consider what can be learnt from this type of programme and which aspects could be embedded into veterinary nursing practice to provide improved support for this group of individuals to make that transition from day one to year one RVN a success.

Preceptorship involves the pairing of an experienced skilled nurse (preceptor) with a new, less experienced nurse (preceptee). Preceptees are novices in a new clinical area and it is important to understand that this not only applies to day one RVNs but also experienced RVNs in a new role or business (Happell 2009; Bott et al. 2011). Preceptorship is different from mentoring as preceptorship has the involvement of a third party who is responsible for the pairing of the experienced nurse with the novice. The professional relationship that is established has the capacity to improve job satisfaction and patient safety because the environment in which the new nurse is working is a safe and supported one. This enables the learning of new skills and the building of confidence and competence within the new clinical environment and role.

Within veterinary nursing there is an established support system in place for student nurses, with a named clinical supervisor supporting students in the clinical workplace and therefore the concept of the next step of 'preceptorship' is not an alien one. In reality, across all veterinary businesses, there will be an induction of sorts for all newly employed staff, including RVNs. Therefore, the word 'preceptorship' may be new but what it is trying to achieve, in terms of a fully integrated safe practitioner working as part of the veterinary team, is not. Having this structure in practice enables the preceptee to work with the preceptor to develop their clinical competencies while maintaining safe practice.

The role of the preceptor can be challenging but it is rewarding, it is also very important in influencing retention rates and job satisfaction (Quek and Shorey 2018). When determining who would make a good preceptor, it is obvious that this would suit someone interested in supporting and teaching others. However, a structured programme to provide preceptors with effective clinical teaching strategies is also valuable. Having this as an ongoing programme of support will ensure that preceptors are kept current regarding the supportive teaching role that they have (Hyrkas and Shoemaker 2007; Haggerty et al. 2012). The other important consideration is the additional workload that the preceptor is taking on, particularly if a formalised skills list is developed for the preceptee to achieve. If this structured supportive role is to be successfully adopted there needs to be consideration made regarding time protected to undertake the preceptorship role. If this is not taken into account, it will lead to poor uptake or engagement with the process by nurses who would otherwise make excellent preceptors (Lewis and McGowan 2015; Tracey and McGowan 2015). A preceptee will not, as they gain these new skills and competencies, provide a full-time equivalent function of a nurse who has been established in the business for some time, but with this early structured support, attrition rates of these new nurses will reduce. Having the preceptor and preceptee on the same shift pattern where possible is a sensible approach for best outcomes (Tracey and McGowan 2015; Quek and Shorey 2018).

New RVNs have the advantage of being in clinical placement for a minimum of 1800 hours prior to registration. However, the transition from student to accountable professional is a challenging one and therefore facilitating that transition though a structured preceptorship programme, would be beneficial. Quek and Shorey (2018) undertook a meta-analysis of literature surrounding this area and they determined that there were key factors that influenced the success of any preceptorship programme, these predominantly focused on the preceptor themselves being prepared for and supported in their role by their manager and for the preceptor to understand the significance of the role for the preceptee and what the factors are that could influence this relationship.

Skills Needed by the Preceptor

The preceptor needs to be familiar with the needs of the preceptee as well as the requirements of the practice in terms of supporting the individual. There needs to be consideration made regarding matching the preceptor and the preceptee; aspects to consider include route of entry into the profession. Within human-centred nursing the difference in qualification level between the preceptee and preceptor resulted in a feeling of being threatened by qualification level (Park et al. 2011), leading to the preceptee being less likely to challenge and question and therefore less likely to learn and understand. There is also a potential risk of this within veterinary nursing with the two routes of entry into the profession (further and higher education).

In addition to linking individuals with the same educational background, other considerations that need to be made include:

- previous experience
- level of competence and confidence
- ability to think critically and reflect
- the establishment of an environment of trust
- the ability to communicate effectively.

The preceptor also needs to be provided with the opportunity to have regular continued professional development related to the preceptorship role (Quek and Shorey 2018), they are often experienced practitioners in a clinical role but are unlikely to have a formal education in clinical teaching (Myrick and Yonge 2005). The importance of the role of preceptor in terms of the transition from day one to year one nurses within the clinical environment and the retention rate cannot be underestimated. Therefore, the establishment of such a role is an important one within veterinary nursing to support early careers nurses in a more formalised way within our profession.

The Challenges of the Role of the Preceptor

There are several challenges to being a preceptor or any other supervisory or training role within veterinary nursing and these will be considered below.

Firstly, there needs to be support for the role by the nursing manager as preceptors are high functioning when this happens. Included in that is a formally reduced patient workload for the preceptor to enable them to focus on their preceptor role. The preceptor also needs to be supported to determine the requirements of the preceptee in terms of skill set development and achievement by setting objectives to meet these. This time spent with the preceptee will help establish what the mutual expectations are and determine the preceptees current abilities and knowledge as well as their previous experience. Having protected time to be able to undertake weekly meetings for review, reflection, and feedback will also facilitate a successful preceptor/preceptee relationship.

Another challenge that is faced in clinical practice is that of the unsafe practitioner (student or RVN). Regardless of the level of the individual, we, as accountable professionals, have a professional commitment to put patient safety at the forefront of everything we do. Therefore, we have to always ask two questions when making a decision regarding the competence of an individual we are working with as clinical supervisor, preceptor, team member, or manager:

1. Would I want this individual caring for one of my animals?
2. Would I want to work alongside this individual as part of the veterinary team?

These are important questions to ask to ensure patient safety as well as the integrity and reputation of the business and the profession. From an ethical standpoint, if the answer of either one of these is no, then the RVN working as the clinical supervisor, preceptor, team member has an obligation to flag the unsafe individual in order that a decision can be made regarding their progression in their role (Earle-Foley et al. 2012).

A human-centred meta-analysis of literature on preceptorship found that when supported in role preparation, reduction of workload and having support from senior leaders, the preceptor role was effective, satisfying, and was paramount in the development in the confidence in nurses transitioning into different roles and areas of responsibility (Ward and McComb 2017). The role of support within veterinary practice is a vital one and helps nurses as they move through the different stages of their careers, the term 'preceptorship' refers to the support of early career nurses but the general principles are applicable in other career transition scenarios.

Summary

This chapter has been written with a view to supporting the clinical nurse educator in their role, in both the classroom and clinic settings. It has provided some insight into how learners learn and what we can do to support that process, and this has included the importance of the alignment of teaching and learning, learning outcomes linked to teaching activities, and assessment for achievement. Consideration of facilitating learning through student-centred active learning techniques enhances the depth of understanding and ensures we produce critical-thinking RVNs.

The transition from student to accountable professional can be made easier by introducing the role of preceptor, and we have a duty to ensure newly qualified professionals are supported in their decision-making in the early part of their career and beyond.

Now visit the companion website where you will find additional resources for this chapter: www.wiley.com/go/badger/professionalism-veterinary-nursing.

References

Akerjordet, K. and Severinsson, E. (2010). The state of the science of emotional intelligence related to nursing leadership: an integrative review. *J. Nurs. Manag.* 18 (4): 363–382.

Albanese, M.A. (2010). Work based learning. In: *Understanding Medical Education: Evidence, Theory and Practice* (ed. T. Swanwick), 37–52. Association for the Study of Medical Education.

Armstrong, P. (2010). *Bloom's Taxonomy*. Vanderbilt University Center for Teaching https://cft.vanderbilt.edu/guides-sub-pages/blooms-taxonomy/ (accessed 24 January 2022).

Austria, M.J., Baraki, K., and Doig, A.K. (2013). Collaborative learning using nursing student dyads in the clinical setting. *Int. J. Nurs. Educ.* 10 (1): 73–80.

Bates, B. (2016). *Learning Theories Simplified. . .and How to Apply Them to Teaching*, 2e. London: Sage Publications.

Benner, P. (1984). *From Novice to Expert; Excellence and Power in Clinical Nursing Practice*. Prentice Hall.

Biggs, J. and Tang, C. (2011). *Teaching for Quality Learning at University*. Maidenhead: Open University Press.

Bloom, B.S., Engelhart, M.D., Furst, E.J. et al. (1956). *Taxonomy of Educational Objectives: The Classification of Educational Goals. Vol. Handbook I: Cognitive Domain*. New York: David McKay Company.

Bott, G., Mohide, E.A., and Lawlor, Y. (2011). A clinical teaching technique for nurse preceptors: the five minute preceptor. *J. Prof. Nurs.* 27 (1): 35–42.

Carpenter, S.K., Witherby, A.E., and Tauber, S.K. (2020). On students' (mis)judgments of learning and teaching effectiveness. *J. Appl. Res. Mem. Cogn.* 9 (2): 137–151.

Christianson, K.L. (2020). Emotional intelligence and critical thinking in nursing students. *Nurse Educ.* https://doi.org/10.1097/NNE.0000000000000801 (Epub ahead of print).

Clarke, P. (2012). Veterinary nursing research: types, importance and dissemination. *Vet. Nurs.* 3 (3): 142–146.

DeSimone, B. (2006). Curriculum design to promote the critical thinking of accelerated Bachelor's degree nursing students. *Nurse Educ.* 31 (5): 213–217.

Dreyfus, S.E. (2004). The five-stage model of adult skill acquisition. *Bull. Sci. Technol. Soc.* 24 (3): 177–181. https://doi.org/10.1177/0270467604264992.

Earle-Foley, V., Myrick, F., Luhanga, F., and Yonge, O. (2012). Preceptorship: using an ethical lens to reflect on the unsafe student. *J. Prof. Nurs.* 28 (1): 27–33.

Erbil, D.G. (2020). A review of flipped classroom and cooperative learning method within the context of Vygotsky theory. *Front. Psychol.* 11: 1157. https://doi.org/10.3389/fpsyg.2020.01157.

Fernandez, R., Salamonson, Y., and Griffiths, R. (2012). Emotional intelligence as a predictor for academic performance in first-year accelerated graduate entry nursing students. *J. Clin. Nurs.* 21 (23–24): 3485–3492.

Gatewood, E., Bromholm, C., Herman, J., and Yingling, C. (2019). Making the invisible visible: implementing an implicit bias activity in nursing education. *J. Prof. Nurs.* 35 (1): 447–451.

Haggerty, C., Holloway, K., and Wilson, D. (2012). Entry to nursing practice preceptor education and support: could we do it better? *Nurs. Prax. N. Z.* 28 (1): 30–39.

Halasa, S., Abusalim, N., Rayyan, M. et al. (2020). Comparing student achievement in traditional learning with a combination of blended and flipped learning. *Nurs. Open* 7 (4): 1129–1138. https://doi.org/10.1002/nop2.492.

Happell, B. (2009). A model of preceptorship in nursing: reflecting the complex functions of the role. *Nurs. Educ. Perspect.* 30 (6): 372–376.

Honey, P. and Mumford, A. (1995). *Using your Learning Styles*. Maidenhead: Peter Honey Publications.

Hyrkas, K. and Shoemaker, M. (2007). Changes in the preceptor role: re-visiting preceptor perceptions of benefits, rewards, support and commitment to the role. *J. Adv. Nurs.* 60 (5): 513–524.

Krathwohl, D.R. (2002). A revision of Bloom's taxonomy: an overview. *Theory Pract.* 41 (4): 212–218. https://doi.org/10.1207/s15430421tip4104_2.

Lewis, S. and McGowan, B. (2015). Newly qualified nurses' experiences of a preceptorship. *Br. J. Nurs.* 24 (1): 40–43.

Long, A. and Lock, B. (2010). Lectures and large groups. In: *Understanding Medical Education: Evidence, Theory and Practice* (ed. T. Swanwick), 139–150. Association for the Study of Medical Education.

Mayer, J.D., Roberts, R.D., and Barsade, S.G. (2008). Human abilities: emotional intelligence. *Annu. Rev. Psychol.* 59 (1): 507–536.

Mezirow, J. (1997). Transformative learning: Theory to practice. *New Directions for Adult and Continuing Education* 74: 5–12. https://doi.org/10.1002/ace.7401.

Miller, G.E. (1990). The assessment of clinical skills/competence/performance. *Acad. Med.* 65: S63–S67.

Morris, C. and Blaney, D. (2010). Work based learning. In: *Understanding Medical Education: Evidence, Theory and Practice* (ed. T. Swanwick), 69–82. Association for the Study of Medical Education.

Myrick, F. and Yonge, O. (2005). Nursing preceptorship: connecting practice and education. *Home Health. Nurse* 23 (10): 680.

Ofqual (2017). Ofqual Handbook: General Conditions of Recognition. https://www.gov.uk/guidance/ofqual-handbook/section-e-design-and-development-of-qualifications#condition-e9-3 (accessed 30 Janiary 2022).

Oxtoby, C. and Mossop, E. (2019). Blame and shame in the veterinary profession: barriers and facilitators to reporting significant events. *Vet. Rec.* 184 (16): 501–502.

Park, J.R., Wharrad, H., Barker, J., and Chapple, M. (2011). The knowledge and skills of pre-registration masters' and diploma qualified nurses: A preceptor perspective. *Nurse Education in Practice* 11 (1): 41–46. https://doi.org/10.1016/j.nepr.2010.06.004.

Parmelee, D.X. and Michaelsen, L.K. (2010). Twelve tips for doing effective Team-Based Learning (TBL). *Medical Teacher* 32 (2): 118–122. https://doi.org/10.3109/01421590903548562.

Petty, G. (2010). *Teaching Today A Practical Guide*, 4e. Nelson Thornes.

Powers, K., Herron, E.K., Sheeler, C., and Sain, A. (2018). The lived experience of being a male nursing student: implications for student retention and success. *J. Prof. Nurs.* 34 (1): 475–482.

Quality Assurance Agency (2014). UK Quality Code for Higher Education: The Frameworks for Higher Education Qualifications of the UK Degree Awarding Bodies. https://www.qaa.ac.uk/docs/qaa/quality-code/qualifications-frameworks.pdf (accessed 27 October 2020).

Quek, G. and Shorey, S. (2018). Perceptions, experiences, and needs of nursing preceptors and their preceptees on preceptorship: an integrative review. *J. Prof. Nurs.* 34 (5): 417–428.

Royal College of Veterinary Surgeons (2014). *Day One Competences for Veterinary Nurses.* London: RCVS. https://www.rcvs.org.uk/document-library/day-one-competences-for-veterinary-nurses (accessed 27 October 2020).

Royal College of Veterinary Surgeons (2016). *Day One Skills for Veterinary Nurses – Small Animal.* London: RCVS. https://www.rcvs.org.uk/document-library/rcvs-day-one-skills-for-veterinary-nurses (accessed 27 October 2020).

Royal College of Veterinary Surgeons (2019). *RCVS Survey of the Veterinary Nursing Profession 2019*. London: RCVS. https://www.rcvs.org.uk/news-and-views/publications/the-2019-survey-of-the-veterinary-nursing-profession (accessed 9 October 2020).

Sam, A.H., Hameed, S., Harris, J., and Meeran, K. (2016). Validity of very short answer versus single best answer questions for undergraduate assessment. *BMC Med. Educ.* 16: 266. https://doi.org/10.1186/s12909-016-0793-z.

Shultz, P. and Baker, J. (2017). Teaching strategies to increase student nurse acceptance and management of unconscious bias. *J. Nurs. Educ.* 56 (11): 692–696.

Souers, C., Kauffman, L., McManus, C., and Parker, V. (2007). Collaborative learning: A focused partnership. *Nurse Educ. Pract.* 7 (6): 392–398.

Süzen, N., Gorban, A.N., Levesley, J., and Mirkes, E.M. (2020). Automatic short answer grading and feedback using text mining methods. *Procedia Comput. Sci.* 169: 726–743. https://doi.org/10.1016/j.procs.2020.02.171.

Tanner, C.A. (2006). Thinking like a nurse: a research-based model of clinical judgement in nursing. *J. Nurs. Educ.* 45 (6): 204–211.

Tracey, J. and McGowan, I. (2015). Preceptors' view on their role in supporting newly qualified nurses. *Br. J. Nurs.* 24 (20): 998–1001.

Victor-Chmil, J. (2013). Critical thinking versus clinical reasoning versus clinical judgement – differential diagnosis. *Nurse Educ.* 38 (1): 34–36.

van der Vleuten, C.P. and Schuwirth, L.W. (2005). Assessing professional competence: from methods to programmes. *Med. Educ.* 39 (3): 309–317. https://doi.org/10.1111/j.1365-2929.2005.02094.x. PMID: 15733167.

Ward, A. and McComb, S. (2017). Precepting: A literature review. *J. Prof. Nurs.* 33 (1): 317–325.

Wood, D.F. (2003). Problem based learning. *BMJ* (Clinical research ed.) 326 (7384): 328–330. https://doi.org/10.1136/bmj.326.7384.328.

Wood, T. (2009). Assessment not only drives learning, it may also help learning. *Med. Educ.* 43 (1): 5–6. https://doi.org/10.1111/j.1365-2923.2008.03237.x. PMID: 19140992.

Wormald, B.W., Schoeman, S., Somasunderam, A., and Penn, M. (2009). Assessment drives learning: an unavoidable truth? *Anat. Sci. Educ.* 2 (5): 199–204. https://doi.org/10.1002/ase.102. PMID: 19743508.

Zhang, J. and Chen, B. (2020). The effect of co-operative learning on critical thinking of nursing students in clinical practicum: A quasi-experimental study. *J. Prof. Nurs.* https://doi.org/10.1016/j.profnurs.2020.05.008.

Examples of Extended Matching Questions

https://global.oup.com/uk/orc/medicine/cox/01student/emqs

Further Reading

Baillie, S., Warman, S., and Rhind, S. (2014). A guide to assessment in veterinary medicine. http://www.bris.ac.uk/vetscience/media/docs/guide-to-assessment.pdf (accessed 6 January 2022).

Benner, P. (1982). From novice to expert. *Am. J. Nurs.* 82 (3): 402–407. https://doi.org/10.2307/3462928.

Cottrell, S. (2001). *Teaching Study Skills and Supporting Learning*. Palgrave.

Lerchenfeldt, S., Mi, M., and Eng, M. (2019). The utilization of peer feedback during collaborative learning in undergraduate medical education: a systematic review. *BMC Med. Educ.* 19 (1): 321. https://doi.org/10.1186/s12909-019-1755-z.

Newton, P.M. and Miah, M. (2017). Evidence-based higher education – is the learning styles 'Myth' important? *Front. Psychol.* 8: 444. https://doi.org/10.3389/fpsyg.2017.00444.

van der Vleuten, C.P. and Schuwirth, L.W. (2019). Assessment in the context of problem-based learning. *Adv. Health Sci. Educ. Theory Pract.* 24 (5): 903–914. https://doi.org/10.1007/s10459-019-09909-1.

Wood, E.J. (2003). What are extended matching sets questions? *Biosci. Educ.* 1 (1): 1–8. https://doi.org/10.3108/beej.2003.01010002.

7 The Role of the RVN in Society

Rebecca Jones

What is Society?

Before considering the role of the RVN within society, we should first consider what 'society' is, its origins and its importance. The term is derived from the Latin 'societas', meaning fellowship, association, or union. Broadly, it can be considered as the organisation of social behaviour and social relationships; the union of a group of people through a prevailing influence, such as cultural or political beliefs. It may be considered an abstract term, having many influences, and, as such, is continuously evolving. A larger, dominant society can also consist of smaller societies, with beliefs or interests at variance with the larger group; these societies are often referred to as a subculture. Individuals will also hold many social roles – within the home, workplace, as part of a professional, religious, or recreational group, for example; so society can also be defined as a web of social roles, the occupants of which interact according to the rules and the knowledge that define these roles (Klüver 2008).

The origins of society are not easy to define but it is generally acknowledged that the social groups of early man were similar to those of other social primates, with the origins of what could be deemed as 'society' beginning with the transition of humans from the nomadic, hunter-gatherer phase to the Neolithic revolution, the development of agricultural settlements and early civilisation. This period formed what sociologists refer to as the pre-industrial period, one of three periods that are considered influential in the development of society as we know it today, the others being the Industrial period and the Post-Industrial period. These periods saw the 'Dawn of Civilisation', the 'Industrial Revolution', and the 'Technological Revolution' and give great insight into how human 'society' has evolved from one akin to other social animals to one with many more complexities; knowledge and invention bringing power and wealth for some, the establishment of social class, political governments, and a more diverse culture which has continued to evolve to this current day.

Throughout history, there have been many sociological theories that attempt to explain the relevance of society. Some believe society is required for stability, regulation, and unification; others believe that society is oppressive and limits our natural

Professionalism and Reflection in Veterinary Nursing, First Edition.
Edited by Sue Badger and Andrea Jeffery.
© 2022 John Wiley & Sons Ltd. Published 2022 by John Wiley & Sons Ltd.
Companion website: www.wiley.com/go/badger/professionalism-veterinary-nursing

development. History has shown that there is truth in both these statements. The subject of the influence of society on the individual and vice versa is commonly debated; does society shape the individual or does the individual shape society? Theorists have expressed strong beliefs in support of both, but it is more widely accepted that they have an interdependent relationship; one grows with the help of the other (Hossain and Korban 2014). A well-balanced society enables the individuals within it to have both dependence and autonomy.

The following are examples of factors that influence the development of society and the individuals within it:

- *Sociocultural influence:* the combination of social and cultural factors – the customs, lifestyles and values – that characterise a society or group.
- *Social stratification:* the way in which people are ranked or ordered – social hierarchy – as a result of socioeconomic influences such as income, education, gender and ethnicity.
- *Social influence:* the way in which individuals change their ideas and actions to meet the needs of a social group or perceived authority.
- *Values and beliefs:* values are our sense of right or wrong, our moral choice. They suggest how individuals/society should behave. Beliefs are the deep-rooted convictions that we hold true, based on our past experiences and not necessarily based on fact. Values and beliefs are an important part of our identity. They are shaped by our sociocultural experiences and social influences.

The complexities of society far exceed the remit of this chapter but having a broad understanding of its relevance, influence and evolution is useful in understanding our own role within it. In addition, it would be remiss not to briefly address the effects of globalisation, advancements in technology, communication, and increased international travel. The often-used term 'global society' is an apt one, given that we are now internationally connected with each other. Many of the issues that we are tackling at a national level are also experienced worldwide, and, as such, require global collaboration.

The devastating effects of the coronavirus pandemic really puts this into context as it serves to remind us of the need to protect ourselves and the world around us, not least the wildlife, domestic and pet species that share the planet with us. The veterinary nursing profession, both within the UK as well as in other countries across the globe, has a role to play in this. RVNs may wish to engage more actively with international projects. At the very least, we should have an awareness of the global context and how this relates to the work that we do.

The Role of the RVN within Society

Based on what we can understand about society, the RVN does not just have one role, we have many. When we become qualified veterinary nurses, we make a declaration to abide by a professional code of conduct; we agree to act according to a professional, legal, and ethical framework. Our professional self is one of the social roles that we fulfil. We will have held many other social roles from birth that will have had great influence on our values, beliefs, and actions, including the decision to become veterinary nurses. We will continue to hold many other social roles, in addition to our professional roles. As veterinary nurses, there is an expectation that we will uphold and apply the values of our profession. As an individual, we also have our own values and beliefs, shaped by our socio-cultural experiences. In our professional and personal lives, we will strive to live by these but there will also be times when our values and beliefs are challenged. Therefore, the first step to understanding our role within society is to understand ourselves – what are the values and beliefs that are important to us and how might these affect our actions? We need to consider our role within society from two perspectives; how we integrate with, and are influenced by, the society in which we live and how, as an individual, we can influence society through advocating our own values and beliefs within our professional and personal lives.

The Veterinary Profession and Society

The first Veterinary School was established in 1760 by Claude Bourgelat, in Lyon, France. Since this time, there have been many societal changes, great and small, that have influenced the veterinary profession. Many of us will recall fondly the tales of James Herriot, but the veterinary practice of this time is barely comparable to the present day.

The most significant changes have occurred in the last 30 years and this is largely attributed to the exponential growth of the companion animal sector. Generational trends have not only resulted in an increase in the numbers of companion animals, they have also contributed to the upgraded status of pets to 'family' for many people. As such, people are more inclined to spend more money on their pets and have much higher expectations for their care. This, in turn, has led to the growth of referral hospitals and veterinary professionals undertaking specialist qualifications within this field. The deregulation of veterinary practices, in 1999, to allow non-veterinary ownership of veterinary practices has been another significant influence; it is estimated that 60–70% of veterinary practices in the UK could be owned by corporate groups by 2027 (Vet Times 2018).

Advancements in technology have been another great influence; the most significant of them being the introduction of the World Wide Web. Since its invention in 1989, the World Wide Web has transformed how people work, live, and communicate, having an impact on every aspect of our lives. The veterinary profession is no exception; the world wide web has radically increased our ability to access up-to-date scientific literature, enabled collaboration for research, given us a global platform for the causes we chose to champion, and much more. It has also provided similar for our clients; they too now have access to a wealth of information and many social platforms to share their views, a progression that may not be so well received by the profession. For the benefits that this technology has delivered, there is also a growing awareness of its pitfalls; notably, the inability to 'disconnect' from this virtual world and the negative influences of social media on mental well-being. However, the online platform really came in to its own during the coronavirus pandemic, enabling the continuation of veterinary care through telemedicine, for example. Other significant technological advancements have been within the field of diagnostics: MRI, ultrasound, digital radiography, and sophisticated anaesthesia monitoring equipment are becoming increasingly commonplace in veterinary practices.

The farming and veterinary industry are closely interlinked; the foot and mouth outbreak in 2001, for example, impacting greatly on both. More recently, the increase in food production, as a result of increasing global population growth, has led to wider challenges; there is growing concern regarding the impacts of this on antimicrobial resistance (AMR), zoonotic disease, ecosystem sustainability, and climate change. The challenges of maintaining global trade, food security, and animal health and welfare have been further complicated by the UK's decision to leave the EU. Factors such as these further highlight the responsibility that the veterinary profession has in the wider society, as a voice for One Health issues and an advocate for animal welfare within this.

Some societal changes occur over time; retention issues within the veterinary profession, as an example, believed to be a result of the changing requirements of the modern-day veterinary professional (Hagen et al. 2020), a shift not just seen within the veterinary profession. Some events are far less subtle and impact on society in ways that we previously could not possibly conceive. As this chapter was being written, the UK was still in the midst of two such events, Brexit and the Coronavirus pandemic.

Animals and Society

Animals have been part of our society from the beginning of civilisation. When we consider the history of human society, it is clear to see how this evolution has influenced our relationship with animals. Our relationship has evolved from a dependency on animals as a food source and means of survival to one where animals are now also depended upon for companionship; integrated into our society as members of our family. It has long been acknowledged that the health of people and animals is interlinked but there is a growing recognition that the interdependency of this relationship extends beyond physical health. Animals share our lives and our living environments; their lives are therefore impacted by societal change as much as our own. The coronavirus pandemic demonstrates just how significant this impact can be.

Prior to the coronavirus pandemic, the growing body of evidence to support the physical and psychological benefits of human-animal interaction was already being promoted under the umbrella of the Human-Animal Bond (HAB). HAB has been identified as having a positive effect on the key indicators of stress and anxiety, leading to improvements in both physical and mental health of the recipients.

The societal shift in recognising that mental well-being is as important as physical health demonstrates how then this shift can impact the lives of animals. The role of dogs assisting people with physical disabilities has existed for years but more recently has expanded to include support for those with behavioural and mental health conditions too. The recognition of the benefits of animal contact has also been embraced by medical healthcare practitioners, with an increased use of animal-assisted therapy in healthcare settings; this instigated the first 'Working Dogs in Healthcare' protocol, published by the Royal College of Nursing (RCN) in 2019.

While there appears no doubt that the HAB can yield many benefits, there clearly is also a need for an element of caution when promoting it. There is a balance to be achieved in supporting the development of this relationship while ensuring that the best interests of both animal and human are also considered. Again, the coronavirus pandemic gives insight into how delicate this balance is. The start of the pandemic saw a significant increase in people looking to purchase pets for companionship, to overcome social isolation. As the situation developed, there arose concerns regarding a surge in behavioural issues, such as separation anxiety, because of pets becoming accustomed to having their owners at home. The economic impact of the pandemic also began to take its toll; at the time of writing, the PDSA had predicted as many as 50 000 more pets being eligible for its services as a result. The pandemic has also seen a boom in puppy sales and an extortionate rise in puppy prices as a result. The strength of the HAB is well publicised, but this bond can also be fragile and often to the detriment of the animal involved.

In addition to the wider societal influence, the dependency of companion animals on their human caregiver means that their lives are also affected by an individual's values, beliefs, and social background. These individual factors, in addition to other factors such as cultural and generational trends, will influence decision-making regarding the purchase of a pet and ultimately dictate the health and welfare of that animal. For example, the decision to purchase a particular dog breed as a status symbol or the decision to feed a pet a raw food diet. These factors can also influence decisions that can have both positive and negative impacts on other species too, the choice to purchase higher welfare meat or to participate in hunting, for example. There are also cultural differences in how animals are viewed, which species are considered food, sacred, unlucky, or sentient, for example.

Society will continue to evolve and along with this, the lives of both people and animals will alter accordingly. We become veterinary nurses to provide care and advocate for animals. Fulfilling this role requires an understanding of the wider society around us and the animals under our care.

Promoting Responsible Pet Ownership

The most recent available literature suggests that 50% of the UK population own a pet, with only 1:5 people undertaking any research before purchasing one (PDSA 2019). A significant number will also underestimate the cost of pet ownership and will have a lack of awareness of the welfare needs of their pet. As discussed, the coronavirus pandemic demonstrates just how impulsive people can be when it comes to purchasing a pet and the potential fallout from such a decision. Positively, though, research demonstrates that education can significantly influence an individual's decision-making and the likelihood of them providing the welfare needs of their pet. Consideration should also be given to extending this education to incorporate the 'pre-purchase' stage of pet ownership; many of the subsequent issues that may be encountered can stem from the lack of knowledge and understanding that leads the owner to purchase an unsuitable species or breed.

As veterinary nurses, we are very familiar with concepts such as the 'five freedoms' and the preventative healthcare recommendations that we should be promoting in support of responsible pet ownership. Broadening this, to help owners understand how their health is intrinsically linked to their pets is also shown to be a motivational factor in their commitment to maintaining their pet's health and well-being (www.habri.org). The animal may be our primary concern, but these interlinks mean that there is a need for us to understand the lifestyle and needs of the owner too, if we wish to ensure better health and welfare for the animal.

One Health and Public Health

The recognition that the health of people and animals is interlinked continues to gain momentum. Initially, the focus was very much on physical health, specifically the ever-present threat of infectious and zoonotic disease. However, there is now recognition that the definition of health is not limited to physical health. Through research, knowledge regarding the comparative factors of human and animal health has also expanded, highlighting further the need for a multidisciplinary and collaborative approach between relevant professions and organisations.

One Health is a concept that aims to promote such an approach, incorporating the health of the environment as well as the health of humans and animals. It recognises that these three components should be considered as a triad; each being intrinsically linked and dependent on each other (Figure 7.1).

Although the umbrella term of One Health is relatively new, the concept itself is not. There have been many references to the interlinks of this triad throughout history. An extension of the One Health concept is One Welfare, which seeks to explicitly recognise the links of animal welfare within this triad, for example the links between animal abuse and human abuse. The Links Group is an organisation that aims to raise awareness of these links through support, training and collaboration with other agencies.

Another initiative of relevance is Public Health, which refers to the organised measures taken to prevent disease, promote health and prolong life in populations as a whole. As with One Health, the principles of Public Health are not new; there are many historical references regarding the role of preventative measures, such as sanitation, in prevention of disease outbreaks and health maintenance. The most

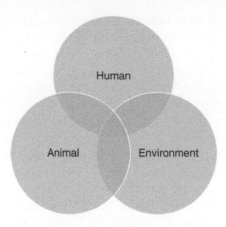

Figure 7.1   One Health triad.

significant of these occurred during the Industrial Revolution; significant migration of people to towns for factory work led to overpopulation, rapid degradation of living environments, and disease outbreaks. Edwin Chadwick, a Social Reformist, published a 'Report on Sanitary Conditions of the Labouring Population', which eventually led to the implementation of the Public Health Act 1848. He recognised the health inequalities between the rich and poor; a topic that is as relevant today as it was then.

The purpose of Public Health remains to protect and improve public health and well-being and reduce health inequalities. Veterinary Surgeons have a long-established role within Public Health; the Veterinary Public Health Association (VPHA) is engaged with the development of national and community legislation, food animal safety and security, zoonotic disease, research and animal welfare and the delivery of animal and public health official controls. Public Health has histori-cally focused on protecting the health of people but it is increasingly recognised that doing this requires a focus on communities as a whole. There is also the suggestion that the definition of 'community' should expand to incorporate all life within this.

Irrespective of what an organisation is called or what is the latest umbrella term to be coined, the fundamental message remains the same; the health of people, animals and the environment is interlinked. The issues of concern in relation to this are as relevant for veterinary nurses as they are for any other healthcare profession.

Examples of One Health/Public Health issues include:

- emerging and re-emerging infectious and zoonotic disease
- antimicrobial resistance
- vaccine hesitancy
- air pollution and climate change
- non-communicable diseases.

As RVNs, we already understand the importance of tackling these issues from the 'animal' perspective. By considering the human/environment components of the triad too, we can impact on these issues at a much wider level. For example, when discussing preventative healthcare for infectious disease, we should expand this discussion to ensure that the owner understands the zoonotic risks of concern. We should also keep up to date with the emerging infectious disease risks and the reasons for example the increased global travel of both people and animals, the trade in exotic pets, and the effects of climate change. The coronavirus pandemic once again highlights the increasing threat of a novel infectious disease and the impact that this has on people, animals, and the environment.

Antimicrobial Resistance (AMR) and vaccine hesitancy are both examples of issues that present a significant global threat. AMR is a naturally occurring process but it is being accelerated by many factors, with inappropriate use being the most significant. Vaccine hesitancy is defined as the reluctance or refusal to be vaccinated and recent data suggests that this is as much a concern for pet vaccination as for humans (PDSA PAWS Report 2019). Education is shown to be key for increasing compliance for both these issues, and this education may also be needed for veterinary professionals; for example, ensuring that our practices are aware of and adhere to, published guidelines regarding antimicrobial use. How these issues are approached with owners is also key, particularly with vaccination hesitancy, if reluctance or refusal is due to being against vaccination on principle. Our role is to provide factual information so that owners can make informed decisions; our role is not to judge or criticise their decisions, however much they may go against our own beliefs. We should also take the time to explore their reasons and not make assumptions; there are many reasons for lack of compliance – misinformation, lack of awareness, cost factors. These issues are great examples of the potential for wider collaboration with other healthcare professionals/organisations; consideration could be given to a joint local campaign to raise awareness within the local community for example.

A non-communicable disease (NCD) is one that is not transmissible from one person/animal to another; examples include cardiovascular disease, respiratory disease, cancer, arthritis, and dementia. Again, these are diseases that RVNs are very accustomed to addressing from the animal perspective, within nurse clinics for example. Both people and companion animals are susceptible to these diseases and there is an increase in research being undertaken to examine the comparative factors of these diseases and their progression in both; notably the similarities and differences between people, dogs and cats. By understanding more about the comparative factors of these diseases in both humans and animals and the influence of their shared living environments and lifestyle choices on these, we again have the potential to apply this knowledge in a way that benefits both humans and animals. Research demonstrates the positive influence of animals on physical and mental health of people but less is known regarding the benefits for the animal in this respect. In fact, the anthropomorphising of pets has been shown to contribute to the likelihood of them acquiring an NCD. For example, there is a link between pet obesity and child obesity; a similar 'co-dependent' relationship existing between pets and owners as for children and parents (Pretlow and Corbee 2016).

The environment, in some ways, can appear to be the 'middle child' within this triad, with interest in this component often stemming from a desire to prevent adverse effects on humans and animals. Environmental changes are often the catalyst for everything else however, so it is vitally important that this component has an equal, if not greater, place at the table. Climate change has been termed the 'threat multiplier', adversely affecting key One Health issues through its impact on the ecological and environmental integrity of living systems (Essack 2018). There is a great opportunity here also for RVNs to extend their role beyond the animals under their care and to take action on environmental issues of concern; reducing our carbon footprint and increasing sustainability. A good first step is signing up to the Investors in the Environment accreditation scheme, in partnership with Vet Sustain.

Understanding the dynamic relationship of all three components within this triad and their influence on each other is key to protecting and improving the health of all.

Public Health supports individuals, organisations and society with addressing health concerns using the framework of the 3 Ps (RCN 2019):

1. Protection – reducing incidence of ill-health through promotion of healthier lifestyles
2. Prevention – surveillance and monitoring of infectious disease, emergency response and vaccination programmes
3. Promotion – health education.

Tannahill's Model of Health Promotion represents these Ps as three overlapping circles, demonstrating the interlinks of these approaches (Figure 7.2). It is another area where new terms supersede old ones but the fundamental principle remains the same; addressing health concerns is not just about one approach. Tannahill's model, in this respect, therefore, remains relevant today.

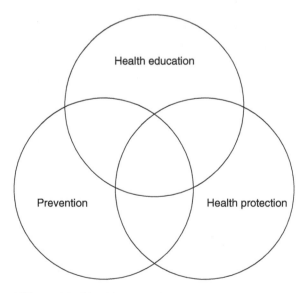

Figure 7.2   Tannahill's model of health promotion.

Tannahill revisited this model in 2008 with the suggestion that the definitions of each of these components could be expanded to include the social, economic, physical, and cultural influences on health, the addressing of health inequalities, and the inclusion of community-led activities, thus promoting the salutogenic approach that is more representative of today's health promotion in human-centred healthcare (Tannahill 2009).

Social determinants of health

Social determinants of health are the conditions in which people are born, live, work, and age; they are the factors mostly responsible for health inequalities seen within and between countries. Measures of socioeconomic status, social integration, and early-life adversity are among the strongest predictors of health and survival outcomes amongst human populations (Snyder-Mackler et al. 2020).

Examples of social determinants of health include:

- living environment
- housing condition
- social connections
- social norms and attitudes
- access to healthcare services
- access to transportation
- availability of community support and recreational activities
- language and literacy
- education
- employment opportunities
- income

There is a direct correlation between levels of income and health status; those with low income are more likely to experience poor health outcomes and are more exposed to health inequalities. Income is also shown to impact on other social determinants of health, for example quality of housing or access to educational opportunities. Far less is known regarding the influence of these factors on animal health, but, given the shared living environments and the companion animal's dependency on their owner, it is reasonable to consider that their health and welfare could be affected by these factors too (Card et al. 2018). There is evidence to suggest that demographic variables, such as geographical location and socioeconomic status, have an influence on the health of animals (Sánchez-Vizcaíno et al. 2017). It is also reported that pet owners in lower deciles of Indices of Multiple Deprivation (IMDs) are significantly less likely to provide preventative healthcare, have pet insurance, and neuter their pet (PAWS Report 2019). Owners of overweight or obese dogs have also been shown to have a lower net income than owners of normal weight dogs (Chandler et al. 2017).

We also know that an owner's individual lifestyle factors can impact on their pet's health; for example, the effects of passive smoking and other health choices, such as diet and physical exercise. Social isolation and loneliness are significant contributing factors to human health, the effects of which are reported to have a comparable effect on health to other factors, such as poor diet and smoking (McNicholas et al. 2005). This is an example of the positive impact of the HAB, with research suggesting that dog ownership, in particular, can enhance social relationships and increase physical exercise (www.habri.org).

Those that feel excluded from society, discriminated against, or live in extreme poverty can be the least likely to access healthcare services, despite often having the worst health (Public Health England: www.gov.uk/government/organisations/ public-health-england). Given the interlinks of the human-animal relationship, we should consider that animal health and animal health inequalities are also affected by the conditions in which animals are born, live, work, and age (Card et al. 2018).

Nursing within the Community

The role of the District or Community Nurse has existed within human-centred nursing since the 1800s. In recent years, there is an increasing need for this type of nursing as patients are discharged from hospital earlier and the elderly population continues to grow. It therefore unsurprising that there appears to be a growing need for a similar role within the veterinary field, one which offers another opportunity for RVNs to reach the wider community. The District or Community Nurse role, in its traditional sense, within the owner's home environment is a valuable one for both pets and their owners. It can help to overcome barriers to accessing healthcare for many different social groups and can also promote a less stressful experience for the animal too. It can also promote social connections for those that are otherwise isolated and provides the opportunity for collaboration with other healthcare professionals, thus promoting the concept of One Health. It is a role that should be approached with due consideration, however. Aside from ensuring that the role can be performed within the remit of current legislation, there are specific issues that come with performing nursing care within the owner's home; lone working and maintaining professional boundaries are examples.

The Queen's Nursing Institute broadly defines 'community nursing as nursing care outside of the acute hospital environment' – in a school, community centre, or general practice, for example. If we apply this definition to our own professional role then the remit for community nursing becomes much broader. There is an opportunity for us to engage with the wider community in a way that includes, but is not restricted to, providing nursing care within the owner's home. Education is shown to be instrumental in making sustained change and could form a significant part of this role. This education needn't be restricted only to our clients, it can, and should, include the extended community – organisations, schools, different social or cultural groups, other healthcare professionals.

As more is understood regarding the parallels between human and animal health, ensuring optimum health and welfare for our patients requires an approach from two perspectives. We need to understand the wider community and the prevailing societal influences *and* understand the factors that are unique to the individual owner and their pet. Having this understanding offers the potential to support both the community and the individual with making sustained changes that will benefit the health and welfare of all. How we approach these changes is also key to our success. There are many initiatives being implemented under the 'patient as a partner' and 'community-centred care' umbrellas within human-centred healthcare. These healthcare approaches focus on the factors that promote and support health and well-being rather than focus on the factors that cause disease. They aim to help establish links between individuals and their wider community. While not all approaches are directly translatable, we can consider how they can be applied in a way that is relevant to veterinary medicine.

Healthcare Approaches

Salutogenesis – an approach that examines the factors contributing to the promotion and maintenance of physical and mental well-being rather than disease, with particular emphasis on the coping mechanisms of individuals which help to preserve health. It is an holistic approach that was first introduced by sociologist, Aaron Antonovsky (Lindström and Eriksson 2005).

Holistic – a system of comprehensive or total patient care that considers the physical, social, economic, spiritual and emotional needs of the patient, his or her response to illness and the effect of the illness on the ability to meet selfcare needs (McFerran 2021).

See also 'Patient-Centred Nursing' below

Community-centred care is a 'whole system' approach which aims to empower individuals with taking control of their health and establishing a greater sense of community through social connections. This type of approach is believed to be an essential way of reducing health inequalities and is particularly effective for vulnerable and marginalised groups.

Social prescribing, sometimes referred to as 'community referral', is the process whereby patients are referred by healthcare professionals or link workers for community support, assisting them with developing skills which will enable them to improve their own health and well-being (RCN 2019).

These approaches recognise that what matters to someone is not the same as what is the matter with them. The latter refers to the patient's clinical needs whereas the former recognises the individual factors and their 'societal perspective'; incorporating these in a way which places value on their involvement as an active participant in their own health and well-being or that of their pets.

Taking action

Public Health England recommends:

1. understanding the local community; what are the different social groups and what are the influences on their health?
2. understanding the impact of the social and emotional needs on health and what affects this – social networks, neighbourhood support, relationships?
3. adopting a patient-centred approach when communicating with individuals
4. finding out what local community and voluntary organisations there are that could help the individual and actively signpost to these.

The growing awareness of both One Health and the influence of social factors is leading to an emergence of collaborative 'community clinics'. In 2018, a joint initiative was undertaken by the PDSA and the NHS to provide health MOTs for both owners and their pets. A study undertaken by Sweeney and Crook (2018) also successfully used a collaborative One Health Community Clinic to overcome barriers and improve access to healthcare; the majority of those attending reporting that they had neither accessed a doctors surgery or a veterinary practice for years. Another study undertaken by Shaw et al. (2008) suggests that veterinary practices should give consideration to the running of 'wellness clinics' as a way to build rapport with owners and their pets and to give dedicated time to explore the social dimensions and lifestyle factors that affect the way they live their lives.

Patient-centred nursing

It could be argued that promoting responsible pet ownership could be driven in a very textbook way; the five freedoms should be adhered to; preventative healthcare should be given. Real life, however, is somewhat different; we cannot simply provide instructions and expect that people can adhere to them. Again, there are many umbrella terms used and different opinions on these approaches, but the fundamental message is that involving the patient (or the client) as a 'partner' in their care can significantly improve health outcomes. This approach is commonly referred to as 'patient-centred care'; focusing care on the whole needs of the individual with consideration and respect for their opinions and assisting them with developing the knowledge and confidence to make informed decisions regarding their health and well-being.

In addition to the parallels between human and animal health, there have been specific links drawn between animal and paediatric health; a similar co-dependant relationship exists between owner and pet as parent and child. Williams and Jewell (2012) therefore suggest that adopting the 'family-centred' approach used within paediatric care is more relevant in its application to veterinary medicine. This requires consideration of the animal and their owner/s as a family unit; understanding that the health and welfare of the animal is dependent on their role within the family and how the family unit functions and lives as a whole.

Understanding and respecting the opinions of the owner is not the same as agreeing with them. The next part of the process is providing them with accurate information in a format that they can understand so that they can make informed choices regarding their pet's health and welfare. The combination of an holistic approach to ascertaining the individual needs plus the provision of the necessary information enables the negotiation and agreement of a healthcare plan that works for all.

The Difference between Compliance and Adherence

We often use the term 'compliance' when referring to whether an owner is following our recommendations. Another term often used synonymously with compliance is 'adherence'. They are, however, subtly different and this is of relevance when considering our approach.

Compliance: refers to the following of instructions or recommendations, for example, 'please give Tiggy one tablet twice a day'; the relationship between the individual and healthcare provider is more autocratic.

Adherence: is the extent to which a person follows an agreed set of actions, as agreed upon between the individual and the healthcare provider; they are partners in decision-making.

Concordance: promotes self-management of health by establishing a relationship of trust between the individual and the healthcare provider, supporting the individual with making the right decision for them, based on their individual health and lifestyle influences.

Adherence and concordance are what we should be aiming for; both are important factors in healthcare outcomes. People that are active in decision-making remain committed to healthcare recommendations for longer; they also gain confidence from implementing a plan that they agree with and understand (Abood 2007).

Health Literacy

Health literacy refers to people having the confidence, skills and knowledge to access and use health information and their ability to navigate healthcare systems. Health illiteracy is recognised as a significant global public health concern; research indicates that 43–61% of English working adults are affected (Public Health England 2015).

Population groups most at risk of limited health literacy are (Public Health England 2015):

- more disadvantaged socioeconomic groups
- people from ethnic minorities
- older people
- people with long-term health conditions
- people with physical or mental disabilities.

While specific groups may be more at risk, it should be acknowledged that health illiteracy can affect everyone at some stage, for example, those that are anxious or distressed when receiving information. We should also be mindful that detecting this issue is not always easy; people may be reluctant to disclose that they have not understood or may not even realise that they have not. It is prudent to consider it as a potential factor during communication.

The NHS Health Literacy Place recommends adoption of the following five approaches to aid patients/clients with understanding the information that is being provided:

1. *Teach back* – confirming that information has been understood by asking owners to 'teach back' the instructions that we have given rather than just saying 'do you understand?'
2. *Chunk and check* – breaking down information into much smaller, manageable chunks and checking understanding using the 'teach back' method before moving on. This technique also gives the opportunity for the owner to ask questions before moving on.
3. *Simplistic language* – we use a range of veterinary terminology and acronyms which owners may not understand, especially if distressed or anxious. We should keep language simple and also consider a terminology handout for the most commonly used terms.
4. *Use of pictures* – pictures, models, diagrams, and other visuals, used to support communication, can be effective in improving understanding.
5. *Offering to assist with paperwork* – we should offer to do this routinely and not just for those owners that we perceive to need help.

Respecting Different Walks of Life

Our society has a growing cultural diversity, due to increasing global connectivity, international travel, immigration and emigration. It is very likely that we will interact with people with different cultural backgrounds; their values, beliefs and customs sometimes being different to our own. In the medical field, research shows that healthcare outcomes are influenced by language or cultural barriers and deep-rooted health-related beliefs. Less is known regarding the impact of this on veterinary healthcare, but it is thought likely to be similar, especially given the added differences in cultural appreciation of the role of animals within society (Mills et al. 2011). Providing optimum care to our patients depends on our ability to communicate our recommendations in a way that can be understood and maintains respect and understanding of the individual's own beliefs.

Culture refers to the beliefs, values, customs, and institutions of ethnic, religious, racial, or social groups; its diversity is one that should be embraced but it is also one that can affect our judgement if we do not fully understand it or it conflicts with our own views. We often refer to being 'non-judgemental' in our decision-making, but the reality is that this can be very hard in some situations. Unconscious bias refers to the way in which we unconsciously assign positive and negative value in our judgement of others, based on our own social-cultural experiences. We can apply this judgement in many different situations – because of a person's age, gender, socio-economic status, or physical and mental capability, for example. These may not be overt, but many of us are likely to apply some form of judgement when initially confronted with certain situations; for example, the likelihood that someone will be able to pay their veterinary bill or the 'neglect' of the obese cat. Occasionally, we will be confronted with a situation that greatly challenges our own values and beliefs. Conscientious objection refers to a strongly held value or belief that an individual could never compromise on (Carvalho et al. 2012). It is possible that we could be confronted with a situation that challenges ours or, conversely, are confronted with an individual who holds their own, for example the refusal of medical treatment on religious grounds.

To be able to appropriately communicate with people from backgrounds that are different to our own, we should first seek to clarify our own beliefs and values. If we do not examine or articulate our own values, we will not be fully effective with our patients (Uustal 1978). We should acknowledge that we do have our own beliefs and are susceptible to bias; these have the potential to affect our decision-making and how we interact with others. Clarifying what these are can help us to pre-empt the situations that we may find challenging. We can extend this further by encouraging team discussion on this subject within our veterinary practices.

In understanding and respecting other walks of life, we need to also ensure that we do not make assumptions. Although certain attributes may be associated with specific cultural groups, for example, not everyone will share the same behaviours and views; each person should be treated as an individual. Likewise, we may make an initial judgement on an individual's circumstances, but we need to ensure that we still ascertain the reality of their situation by engaging in open-ended dialogue and active listening. For example, although there is a correlation between socioeconomic factors and reduced preventative healthcare, the assumption should not be made that this is financially driven; it may be due to a lack of knowledge.

Cultural competency refers to a set of congruent behaviours, attitudes and policies that come together in a system or among professionals to enable effective work in cross-cultural situations (CDC).

We can develop our veterinary practice's cultural competence and awareness of other social backgrounds by:

- inter-team discussion – discussing our own cultural views and experiences, our individual values and beliefs and any potential barriers that we foresee
- gaining knowledge of our local community – its demographics and socio-cultural make-up
- reaching out to different social groups and organisations.

Future Generations of Society

Child development is a dynamic process with many influences, including parental relationships, social networks, and other economic and social conditions. The relationship between children and animals is still a relatively new area of research but there is consistent evidence to indicate that this relationship can also be influential in a child's development (Endenburg and vanLith 2011).

Attachment to pets can promote social development, social competence, and increased social interaction and communication (Purewal et al. 2007). Research also indicates positive development of self-esteem and empathy for others (Endenburg and vanLith 2011). These benefits are not just seen through pet ownership; interactions with animals through other means, such as within the school classroom, have also been shown to be beneficial (Kotrschal and Ortbauer 2003). However, as with the HAB generally, research regarding the benefits and enjoyment for the animals involved is lacking (The Dogs Trust: www. dogstrust.org.uk) and so caution should be applied in promoting child-animal interaction without careful consideration for the potential negative implications.

Children are the next generation of pet owners; learning how to behave around animals can teach them responsibility, empathy, and respect for animals and others (Figure 7.3). These are important life skills and, as such, there is a growing call for education on animal welfare to form part of the school curriculum. There is now a wealth of educational programmes available for children, mainly provided by the larger animal charities; the PDSA, Blue Cross, RSPCA, and The Dogs Trust all have educational programmes and free resources available for schools.

Programmes available include:

- *PDSA Petwise Award* – a curriculum linked programme aimed at primary-aged children on the five welfares of pets
- *The Dogs Trust Understanding Dogs Workshops* – workshops to promotes safe behaviour around dogs
- *RSPCA Generation Kind* – several projects aimed at nurturing kindness and compassion towards animals.

Education for children is incredibly important but, given that their parental relationships also have great influence on their development, this education should also be extended to include the wider family. Given the high likelihood that animals will also be present in the household before the arrival of a child, this education should also seek to capture expectant parents. Again, there are a wealth of resources available to assist with this.

Examples of how RVNs can play a role in the education of children and their extended families:

- signposting to appropriate resources
- setting up educational nurse clinics

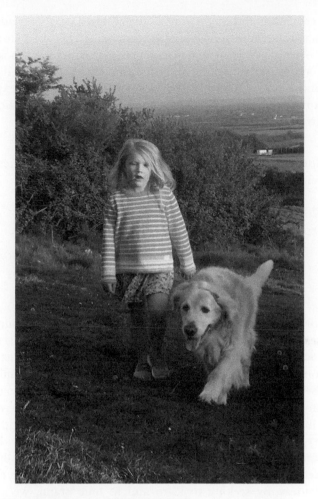

Figure 7.3   Relationship between child and animal.

- supporting Raise Awareness Campaigns within our practice
- speaking within our local community – schools, local organisations, community events
- writing articles or having a blog in a local newspaper/social media page.

Examples of topics:

- animal welfare
- preventative healthcare
- education regarding pet ownership – selecting the right pet, associated costs, pet needs
- integrating a new baby and pet
- safe behaviour around pets
- the HAB and One Health interlink.

Providing education and opportunities for children or young adolescents need not be restricted to companion animals. Extending this to include the natural environment – nature, wildlife, environment – can also have a positive effect on their mental and physical well-being and, again, they are more likely to have a connection and show empathy if they have an opportunity to experience it. As with educational resources on companion animal care, there are several charities that offer outreach projects and resources to support this:

- the Wildlife Trusts – Wildlife Watch, Wild School Award, Forest Schools and family events
- National Trust
- RSPB – Wild Challenge
- David Sheppard Wildlife Foundation – school visits.

Voluntary Work

Voluntary work provides another opportunity for us to use our nursing skills and support causes that we feel passionate about. Opportunities in this sector are vast and extend locally, nationally, and globally. They provide an opportunity for us to experience something outside of our employed roles; an opportunity to combine both the skillset of our professional roles and our own individual interests. Although there are many animal charities that we may wish to support, we needn't restrict ourselves to just this sector. We can also consider involvement with charity work or community projects as a way to expand our knowledge of wider society and the issues faced. Voluntary work of this description can be a really good way to gain a balanced perspective and ascertain the reality of a situation, rather than our preconceived ideas. By seeking to learn and to understand, we can unlock the potential for us to help in a way that supports the concept of One Health. There are already many incredible voluntary organisations that exist because of this mindset – Street Vet, Mission Rabies, The Links Group, and Vet Sustain, to name just a few.

Not all of us may be able to devote significant time to support charities such as these but there are other ways that we can still get involved. We may consider choosing a charity that we wish to support as a practice or perhaps inviting a charity group to come and speak with the team, to promote a better understanding of the work that they do. Examples of such work may include 'Dementia UK' or 'Scope UK' – understanding the impact of dementia on a person and how we can support them with caring for their pets or how we can better support equality for those with disability.

We can also consider applying for a trustee role within a charity; these roles are responsible for the management and administration of the charity organisation and can enable us to have a voice regarding the direction and focus of the charity's work.

Summary

In the same way that Veterinary Nurses are not Veterinary Surgeons, neither are we human-centred nurses. We need to acknowledge that we have a professional and legal framework that we need to work within and we should be careful not to overstep these boundaries. However, we also need to recognise that expanding our knowledge wider than just the health and welfare of the animals under our care is relevant and important to us as professionals in our own right.

Our role in society is a combination of understanding what society needs from us but also how our own values and beliefs connect with this – what are the issues that we feel passionately about and what do we want to advocate for? When might our values and beliefs be challenged and may we overcome this by seeking to learn and understand?

The One Health concept is dynamic and constantly evolving. Understanding of the impact of social and cultural factors on the health and well-being of people is widely recognised and has driven a change in approach for human-centred healthcare. Less is known regarding the impact of these factors on animal health and well-being but, given the interlinks of the One Health triad and the close relationship of the HAB, it is becoming apparent that these factors should also be considered relevant to veterinary healthcare. In addressing the health issues of animals and people, we should also remember that the One Health concept represents a triad, which includes the health of the environment; the fundamental message is that we are all connected.

The coronavirus pandemic has been a wake-up call to just how connected we all are and just how significantly an event can alter the course of society. With this in mind, we should consider whether it is just a 'role' that Veterinary Nurses hold in society, or whether we should consider it more of a 'responsibility'.

References

Abood, S.K. (2007). Increasing adherence in practice: making your clients partners in care. *Vet. Clin. North Am. Small Anim. Pract.* 37 (1): 151–164.

Card, C., Epp, T., and Lem, M. (2018). Exploring the social determinants of animal health. *J. Vet. Med. Educ.* 45 (4): 437–447.

Carvalho, S., Reeves, M., and Orford, J. (2012). Relating your values, morals and ethics to nursing practice. *Indep. Nurse* 2012 (2): https://doi.org/10.12968/indn.2012.20.2.89815.

Chandler, M., Cunningham, S., Lund, E.M. et al. (2017). Obesity and associated comorbidities in people and companion animals: a one health perspective. *J. Comp. Pathol.* 156 (4): 296–309.

Endenburg, N. and vanLith, H. (2011). The influence of animals on the development of children. *Vet. J.* 190 (2): 208–214.

Essack, S. (2018). Environment: the neglected component of the one health triad. *Lancet Planet. Health* 2 (6): 238–239.

Hagen, J.R., Weller, R., Mair, T.S., and Kinnison, T. (2020). Investigation of factors affecting recruitment and retention in the UK veterinary profession. *Vet. Rec.* 187: 354.

Hossain, A. and Korban, A. (2014). Relationship between individual and society. *Open J. Soc. Sci.* 2: 130–137.

Klüver, J. (2008). The socio-cultural evolution of our species. *EMBO Rep.* 9: 55–58.

Kotrschal, K. and Ortbauer, B. (2003). Behavioral effects of the presence of a dog in a classroom. *Anthrozoös* 16 (2): 147–159.

Lindström, B. and Eriksson, M. (2005). Salutogenesis. *J. Epidemiol. Community Health* 59: 440–442.

McFerran, T.A. (2021). *A Dictionary of Nursing*, 8e (ed. E.A. Martin and J. Law). Oxford: Oxford University Press.

McNicholas, J., Gilbey, A., Rennie, A. et al. (2005). Pet ownership and human health: a brief review of evidence and issues. *BMJ* 331: 1252.

Mills, J., Volet, S., and Fozdar, F. (2011). Cultural awareness in veterinary practice: student perceptions. *J. Vet. Med. Educ.* 38 (3): 288–297.

PDSA (2019). PDSA Animal Wellbeing (PAW) Report 2019. https://www.pdsa.org.uk/what-we-do/pdsa-animal-wellbeing-report/past-reports (accessed 3 February 2022).

Pretlow, R. and Corbee, R. (2016). Similarities between obesity in pets and children: the addiction model. *Br. J. Nutr.* 116 (5): 944–949.

Public Health England (2015). *Local Action on Health Inequalities: Improving Health Literacy to Reduce Health Inequalities*. London: Public Health England.

Purewal, R., Christley, R., Kordas, K. et al. (2007). Companion animals and child/adolescent development: a systematic review of the evidence. *Int. J. Environ. Res. Public Health* 14 (3): 234.

Royal College of Nursing (2019). Working with Dogs in Health Care Settings. https://www.rcn.org.uk/professional-development/publications/pub-007925 (accessed 3 February 2022).

Sánchez-Vizcaíno, F., Noble, P.J.M., Jones, P.H. et al. (2017). Demographics of dogs, cats, and rabbits attending veterinary practices in Great Britain as recorded in their electronic health records. *BMC Vet. Res.* 13: 218.

Shaw, J.R., Adams, C.L., Bonnett, B.N. et al. (2008). Veterinarian-client-patient communication during wellness appointments versus appointments related to a health problem in companion animal practice. *J. Am. Vet. Med. Assoc.* 233 (10): 1576–1586.

Snyder-Mackler, N., Burger, J., Gaydosh, L. et al. (2020). Social determinants of health and survival in humans and other animals. *Science* 368 (6493): eaax9553.

Sweeney, J. and Crook, P. (2018). Clinical one health: a novel healthcare solution for underserved communities. *One Health* 6: 34–36.

Tannahill, A. (2009). Health promotion: the Tannahill model revisited. *Public Health* 123 (5): 396–399.

Uustal, D. (1978). Values clarification in nursing: application to practice. *Am. J. Nurs.* 78 (12): 2058–2063.

Vet Times (2020). Big 6: rising corporatisation. www.vettimes.co.uk/article/big-6-rising-corporatisation/ (accessed 3 February 2022).

Williams, D. and Jewell, J. (2012). Family-centred veterinary medicine: learning from human paediatric care. *Vet. Rec.* 170: 79–80.

8 The Reflective Practitioner

Sue Badger

What is Reflection and Why is it Important?

Collins English Dictionary (1988) attributes no less than five definitions to the word 'reflection', ranging from 'the image of an object given back by a mirror' to 'conscious thought or meditation' (p. 415). Within the framework of this chapter, the latter definition is most appropriate, but it is useful to consider the former image, as the purpose of reflection in this context is to encourage practitioners to reflect thoughts and emotions so that a deeper level of knowledge and understanding is obtained.

Put simply, reflection is a process that enables the individual to make sense of an experience by viewing it from a new perspective, which enables a deeper understanding. Reflection has been a cornerstone of nursing practice for many years, and it is generally viewed as a useful tool that can assist student nurses to learn from their practical experience as well as a means of helping qualified nurses to provide optimum care and support for their patients, (Jootun and McGarry 2014; Caldwell and Grobbel 2013).

Within the context of veterinary nursing, the use of reflection can aid in the development of both professional and personal insight, which has the potential to impact and improve clinical practice and enhance patient welfare. It is therefore a 'given' that reflection should be a cornerstone of exemplary nursing practice; or should it? As a natural reflector, this author would personally advocate its use; however, there are a number of criticisms that should be explored by anyone considering engaging with the process. These include the fact that, whilst reflection is a natural process for many people, for others it is not easy to adopt the mindset required to participate effectively and this will pose a significant barrier, especially where reflection is a requirement, for example as part of professional development planning (PDP).

The necessity of including a personal dimension in the reflective activity also requires the management of a safe and supportive environment, especially where reflective narratives may be aired publicly, for example in a reflective group scenario.

Professionalism and Reflection in Veterinary Nursing, First Edition.
Edited by Sue Badger and Andrea Jeffery.
© 2022 John Wiley & Sons Ltd. Published 2022 by John Wiley & Sons Ltd.
Companion website: www.wiley.com/go/badger/professionalism-veterinary-nursing

If this safe and confidential environment is not well managed, the potential effect on vulnerable participants can be detrimental. Brookfield (1993) described the possibility of less confident individuals feeling pressured into presenting a 'false self' within a reflective group scenario in order to appear fully confident and competent practitioners. Meaningful reflection must, by its nature, be truthful in order to be effective.

It could also be argued that reflection is more suited to an andragogical model of learning in that the 'expert' nurse possesses a greater wealth of experience and self-awareness than the student or newly qualified nurse and is therefore more comfortable with the concept of exploring both the emotive elements and the less positive learning experiences. This is significant with respect to the implementation of personal development planning for student nurses, who are primarily young individuals, sometimes with little experience of life and limited personal insight. PDP will only work if participants view it as an integral part of their own learning journey and can appreciate the benefits that it brings to their ability to make sense of the process. To enable this to take place they (and their mentor/clinical coach) must view reflection as a normal element of the learning process as a whole and it should become second nature for both students and mentors alike. Therefore, the clinical environment or learning institution must implement reflective practice as policy and ensure that it is embedded into the day-to-day life of everyone involved. This can pose a significant hurdle within a very busy clinical environment and can lead to resistance to its adoption by mentors and students alike.

Theory of Reflection

The importance of reflection as an integral part of deeper learning was first advocated by Dewey (1933), who argued that the ability of an individual to reflect is initiated by the identification of a problem and the uncertainty that is generated by that problem. He further suggested that to successfully reflect, the individual must bring their beliefs and assumptions to bear. Dewey's progressive viewpoint made a unique impact on education and had a significant influence on other educational researchers. Dewey ascribed five stages to the reflective learning process:

1. Suggestions, in which the individual works towards possible solutions.
2. An intellectualisation of the difficulty or perplexity that has been felt (directly experienced) and translation into a problem to be solved.
3. The use of one suggestion after another as a leading idea, or hypothesis, to initiate and guide observation and other skills in collection of factual material.
4. The mental expansion of the idea, or assumption of a supposition, by means of a reasoned approach to the issue.
5. Testing the hypothesis by overt or imaginative action.

Dewey (1933)

However, Dewey's somewhat mechanistic approach did not allow for the influence of the emotional and behavioural perspective on the learning process and as a consequence. Boud et al. (1985) used Dewey's model as the precursor to their three-stage approach.

Returning to the Experience

The individual 'plays back' the experience mentally and in doing so considers the details and thus gains a new awareness or insight of the situation, this enables the gaining of a new perspective. However, the process may be constrained by the feelings evoked by the replaying of the experience and it is essential that these should be identified and acknowledged in order for the reflective process to be successful. This can be very difficult for the novice, who may have to deal with a variety of circumstances during their learning journey that are often painful to recall due to their nature.

Attending to Feelings

It follows that the experience will generally be more rewarding if it and the outcome were both positive. Boud et al. (1985) suggested that a positive affective state of mind would enable the pursuit of both cognitive learning and emotional growth.

Conversely, negative feelings may act as powerful barriers to the process of reflection and learning and must be identified and placed in perspective. This may be difficult, especially where the individual is lacking in confidence and is reviewing a negative experience.

Re-evaluating the Experience

This stage consists of four elements; *association*, that is, the connection of the new information to that which is already known by the individual, followed by the formulation of relationships between the new and the known, termed *integration*. This is followed by *validation* of the information and then *appropriation* of the knowledge as belonging to the individual. Boud et al. (1985) considered that these steps are elements of a whole, rather than discrete stages, through which the individual passes in a well-defined order.

Donald Schön (1987) described professional everyday practice as complex and not easily understood through technical rational models. He referred to this everyday practice as 'the swampy lowlands' of practice, i.e., everyday practice is messy, unpredictable, complex, challenging, and stressful. Consequently, the professional practitioner needs to develop ways of understanding the everyday world in order to learn from clinical practice.

In a move away from propositional knowledge, that is, learning about factual information and technical skills, Donald Schön coined the term 'Reflective Practice' to describe the processes that experienced versus inexperienced engineers used, to engage with the reflective part of the learning experience in a professional context. Schön suggested that factual knowledge alone is of limited value for the student because it does not take into account the reality of the everyday issues that the student will experience in the workplace. Therefore there is a need to build upon the underpinning knowledge previously gained in the classroom with experiential knowledge, which is acquired when the emerging professional undertakes the practical work-based part of their training, during which time they engage with the skills required and have the opportunity to observe and engage with experienced practitioners. Reflection enables them to integrate the theory with the real world and make sense of it. This continues when they become qualified professionals, as learning does not end when they cease being students. Patricia Benner (1984) described a five-stage continuum from Novice to Expert based upon the Dreyfus Model of Skills Acquisition. This theory also provides a useful reminder that an individual continues to learn and hone professional ability and insight, and indeed this does not end once they reach the expert stage!

Schön proposed a new epistemology of practice in which the experienced practitioner recognises and responds to a new situation or problem (Reflection-in-Action) using previous experience and understanding (Knowledge–in-Action). He contrasted this with what he termed 'Reflection-*on*-Action', which is a retrospective contemplation of professional practice undertaken by an inexperienced individual. This process enables the individual to analyse the experience and in doing so to uncover the additional realities inherent in the practice.

Knowing-in-action is the unconscious, intuitive knowing or 'know how': When we have learned how to do something, we can execute smooth sequences of activity, recognition, decision, and adjustment without having, to consciously 'think about it'. Think of a common skill that most people learn in life, for example learning to drive. When first learning to drive, conscious thought must be given to every aspect of the process, but once learned by dint of repetition, these become second nature and the driver no longer has to consciously think about the individual steps.

Our spontaneous knowing-in-action usually gets us through the day. However, sometimes a familiar routine may produce an unexpected result, or it may not be possible to solve a problem using the usual strategies. Sometimes, even if the problem has been solved, there is something unusual about the result. In such situations, practitioners can either ignore the incident, or choose to reflect upon it. Repetitive practice may lead to problems such as no longer questioning the assumptions that underpin practice. Performing a task in a particular manner because it's the way it was initially taught, and it has never been questioned (unless an individual is prepared to take a self-challenging stance), would be the most common example of this non-questioning approach. Evidence-based practice (EBP) is one strategy that is used to challenge these assumptions. Thus, knowing-in-action alone may lead to missed opportunities to reflect and learn from experiences.

Reflection-in-action occurs at a time when you can still make a difference to the particular practice situation, i.e. its 'on-the-spot' reflection. You may be surprised by an event in practice such as an unexpected outcome, either pleasant or unpleasant, and find that your normal practice is interrupted by an immediate reflective response, that is, you are thinking about what you are doing as you do it. Reflection-in-action has a critical function of questioning the assumptions that underpin knowing-in-action. It gives rise to on-the-spot experimentation because of our awareness and observation of new phenomena that occur in our clinical practice.

Reflection-on-action is undertaken after the event. This approach can be applied to the process that students engage with as part of their learning. Their lack of experience in the workplace means that they have little to refer to when contextualising new experiences and are still unfamiliar with reflection as a skill: therefore they are compelled to reflect retrospectively.

Reflection-on-action has also been widely applied in nursing practice and nursing curricula through a variety of approaches, such as reflective writing which involves the use of a narrative approach, group reflection, and critical incident analysis. A learning diary is, at least in part, a reflective diary too, as making notes in in the diary involves the process of reflection-on-action provided the right mindset is adopted.

Clegg (2004) and others have cast some doubt on Schön's concepts; however, they do agree that reflective practice does formalise the differentiation between the purely technical approach practised by the novice and the artistry adopted by the expert practitioner. The latter individual is able to reflect-in-action and in doing so can alter their practice according to the particular set of circumstances encountered at the time. In other words the expert RVN will have the underpinning knowledge and skill-base to enable a flexible approach that increases the potential for successful responses to emergency situations in the workplace – it could be said that they are able to think on their feet!

Clegg and Bradley (2006) surveyed two groups of educators who undertook different continuous professional development (CPD) packages and compared the different approaches to reflection that the students adopted. They found that, as predicted by Schön, the more experienced students in the first group approached reflection in a more abstract manner whilst the less experienced students required guidance in the form of set reflective tasks to enable them to gain an insight into the ethos of reflection.

Larrivee (2008) described a number of levels of reflection in student teachers, from pre-reflection, where the teacher is primarily reactive, to classroom situations and surface reflection is primarily confined to tactical issues, to pedagogical reflection where the teacher's goal is to improve practice and engage with the students. Finally, critical reflection occurs when the teacher has progressed to a level of accomplishment whereby it becomes possible to engage with self-reflection and philosophical ideologies

Agyris and Schön (1974) explored the relationship between theory and the consequences of action when put into practice. Agyris believed that everyone has a mind map of how to deal with specific actions and will tailor underpinning theory to support this understanding and probable outcome. In this way, we can rationalise our behaviour based upon our understanding of normal responses to specific circumstances, so-called congruence. If this does not happen as we expect, we can use a reflective mindset to understand why our preconceived outcome did not arise. His significant body of research (much of it with Donald Schön) gave rise to the development of models of single- and double-loop learning.

Jasper (2003) described reflective practice as having three components in the form of a reflective cycle:

- experiences that happen to an individual
- the reflective processes that take place in order to enable the individual to learn from those experiences
- the resultant action that occurs when new perspectives are gained of the experiences.

Whilst it is not argued that reflection is more important than the other stages of the learning process, a number of educationalists have emphasised the role that reflection appears to play in enhancing it. Experts such as Dewey and Schön have stated that superficial learning, which involves the memory alone, can take place without reflection; but for deeper learning to take place, reflection has to form part of the process.

Kolb's experiential learning cycle (see Figure 8.1) demonstrates in greater detail, the integral part that reflection appears to play in the learning experience. Although this cycle may be entered at any stage it can be seen that the ability to 'take stock' of the experience, be it reflection upon the content of a lecture or an experience

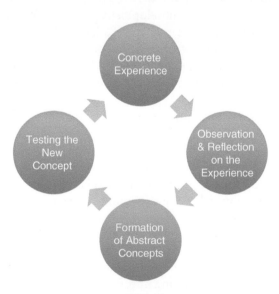

Figure 8.1   Kolb's four-stage model of learning. Source: Based on Kolb 1984/Prentice Hall.

within a vocational context, enables the individual to 'make sense' and to learn from the experience.

However, Wallace (1996) argued that Kolb does not consider how the experiential learning transfers from a 'remote' (e.g. classroom) experience to the real thing. He suggested that a training experience that is divorced from the job could never be more than a valuable supplement to the vital 'hands on' experience of learning to do the real thing.

The Use of Reflection in the Student Learning Environment

The work of educational researchers such as Kolb (1984) and Honey and Mumford (1992) explored the learning process from the perspective of the individual student and their requirements for successful learning. This work contributed to the design of 'taxonomies of learning', which in general place a much greater emphasis on the delivery of learning by means of different teaching techniques that suit the individual learner's needs and a change in methodology where the student is the centre of the process rather than the passive recipient, as in the more traditional didactic approach.

Brockbank and Ian (1998) referred to the concept of dialogue as an essential element of reflection, both internal dialogue, which facilitates personal insight, and the need for external dialogue with one or more colleagues in order to receive feedback and to evaluate the reflective process. They also described the early research on the subject of how learning takes place as being driven by behavioural and cognitive psychology. Outcomes were required to be observable, and as such the focus was on measuring the student's intellectual output. Factors such as previous learning and experience were considered to be variables, which could not be measured and were thus unimportant. The process of learning was seen as a passive one on the student's part and the emphasis was on the regurgitation of factual information. Nowadays, with the help of learning taxonomies, learning is viewed as part of a process that enhances the individual's life experience by recognising and developing their potential. Terms such as 'lifelong learning' and 'transitional learning' are now used to describe the philosophy that learning takes place continuously in all facets of life and is not confined to an individual's school, college, or university experience.

The issue of reflective learning is complicated by the fact that the term is used as both an essential part of the cognitive learning process, as defined by Dewey and Boud, as well as an integral element of the process of learning new skills and honing existing ones within a professional context, for example within the teaching and nursing professions. This is underlined by the fact that within the academic environment the term PDP has been used to refer to *Personal* Development Planning in some sectors whereas it is used to refer to *Professional* Development Planning by regulatory bodies such as the Royal College of Veterinary Surgeons (RCVS). The reality is that any reflective activity must, by its nature, involve both elements in order to facilitate meaningful learning.

Reflection in the Professional Context

As has already been described, there is a range of models of reflection available that can be implemented to engage with the concept. Whichever framework is used, it should be implemented in such a way that it is accessible and its use is not onerous.

In veterinary nursing, individual reflection is the most commonly used approach and can be facilitated in a variety of ways including learning journals/reflective diaries, an online app which enables either a written or verbal report to be entered, as well as additional resources such as appropriate images or additional recorded files of discussion with colleagues and peers. It is important to be aware of the context when recording images and third-party input with respect to confidentiality and, if necessary, anonymity. The RCVS 1CPD tool should be embraced by RVNs as a means of engaging with reflective practice.

Paired reflection can take the form of a narrative that takes place between two colleagues, most often a less experienced individual and a more senior colleague such as a mentor or preceptor. This can also be recorded by mutual agreement and returned to for further discussion at a later date as necessary. It opens up the opportunities for a more objective stance on the reflective process by virtue of the additional perspective and enables fruitful discussion to take place based upon these new perspectives. It must take place in a supportive environment and the reflector must feel comfortable with the process in order for it to be a useful exercise that is positive and enlightening.

Group learning might be considered the next step up from paired reflection but it should be viewed as a significant one as the interaction within a reflective group can be much more dynamic due to the number of different viewpoints that will be brought to bear. For this reason group sizes should be small and it is even more important that clear guidelines are given regarding the need to build a supportive and non-judgemental environment. Benefits include:

- a range of different perspectives are offered that are driven by greater objectivity
- points can be raised that the reflector would not have considered and these enable new questions to be asked and new conclusions reached
- different levels of knowledge and experience are brought to the discussion which can facilitate a change in the reflector's understanding.

The group can be formed of different individuals depending upon the focus of reflection and falls into three main categories, for example, work colleagues, friends or peer group members and professional staff such as lecturers, link tutors, or more senior members of the practice team. In addition, groups can be made up of disparate individuals from each of the groups above and this has the benefit of enabling a wide spectrum of viewpoints to be brought to the discussion. It is important that the group facilitator is aware of the group dynamics and conscious that each group has its own potential risks, for example, the reflector will feel more comfortable reflecting in a group of peers than in a group composed of senior staff members, but each group has its own inherent advantages.

There are myriad templates and frameworks that can be implemented for reflection within the workplace and it would be impossible to cover them all within the space allowed for this chapter. Most employ the common approach of cyclical or spiral progression from experience to reflection and resolution.

Borton's Development Framework (1970)

This three-stage framework is of particular relevance for novice practitioners because of its simple approach to reflection within the clinical environment, which takes the form of a series of questions:

Question	Examples	Purpose
What?	*What* was I doing? *What* events led up to the incident?	Identification of the experience and breaking it down into its components.
So What?	*So, what* information would enable me to understand what happened? *So, what* might I have done differently?	Exploration of the different components of the experience to enable an understanding to be reached. This may involve drawing on previous experiences as well as existing or new knowledge.
Now What?	*Now What* do I think I should do to ensure that I don't find myself in that situation again? *Now What* can I learn from the experience? *Now What* additional information do I need to help me improve my ability to manage the situation in future?	Having analysed the experience, the individual can plan a suitable action or intervention in either a personal or professional context depending upon the nature of the experience.

(Borton 1970)

By working through these stages in a logical manner, the individual can make sense of the incident or experience and gain a deeper level of understanding and insight with a potential change in practice as a result.

Gibbs (1988) takes a similar approach but in a cyclical manner (Figure 8.2), and the focus is on the affective domain, which means that this can be a powerful tool to use where reflection is aimed at making sense of the reflector's emotional response to an incident or experience.

Stephenson's approach (Stephenson and Burns 1994) broadens the range of reflection to include others as well as broader issues, including the ethical dimension.

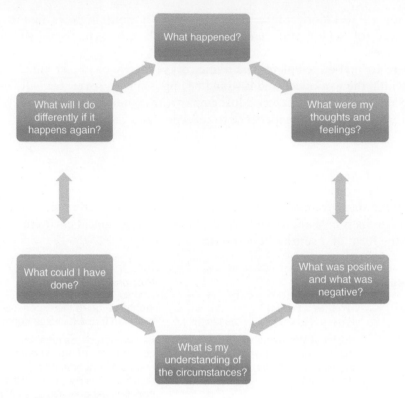

Figure 8.2   Gibbs' cyclical approach.

Choose a situation from your experience. Ask yourself. . .

- What was my role in this situation?
- Did I feel comfortable or uncomfortable? Why?
- What actions did I take?
- How did I and others act?
- Was it appropriate?

- How could I have improved the situation for myself, my colleagues?
- What can I change in future?
- Do I feel as if I have learnt anything new about myself?

- Did I expect anything different to happen? What and why?
- Has it changed my way of thinking in any way?
- What knowledge from theory and research can I apply to this situation?
- What broader issues, for example ethical, political, or social, arise from this situation?
- What do I think about these broader issues?

(Stephenson and Burns 1994)

John's Model of Structured Reflection (1995)

Based on the work of Carper (1978), John's model uses 'cue' questions to reduce an experience or incident into steps with the use of a number of reflective questions:

Identify the incident and put it into context	Describe the experience What essential factors contributed to this experience? What were the significant background factors to this experience?
Reflection	What was I trying to achieve? Why did I act as I did? What were the consequences of my action for those involved including the client, colleagues, myself, others? How did I feel about this experience when it was occurring? How did the client feel about it? How did I know how they felt about it? What factors influenced my decisions and action? What knowledge influenced my decisions and action?
Alternative Action	Could I have dealt differently with the situation? What others choices of action did I have? What would be the consequences of these other choices of action?
Learning	How do I now feel about this experience? Could I have dealt better with the situation? What have I learned? • Ethical – moral challenges • Clinical – the science of veterinary nursing • Aesthetics – the art of veterinary nursing • Personal – insight How will this change my future practice?

(adapted from Johns 1995)

Goodman's Levels of Reflection

Goodman (1984) suggests that there are three levels of reflection that may be achieved by a reflective practitioner:

First level	Reflection to reach objectives using personal aims which may be set by the practitioner or aims set by the tutor in the case of an inexperienced student
	Criteria are superficial in that they relate to easily identifiable goals such as effectiveness and accountability
Second level	Reflection on the relationship between pre-set principles, which may be influenced by experience, cultural values, and knowledge. An understanding of the specific consequences of particular actions is gained through reflection at this level and applied to professional practice
Third level	Reflection that incorporates and builds upon the previous levels to enable the individual to appreciate the 'bigger picture' which may involve placing the reflection within a wider social, moral/ethical, and cultural context in order to gain deeper insight and draw more meaningful outcomes.

(based on Goodman 1984).

The inexperienced reflector will focus on the initial level in order to develop a narrative of the incident or circumstance that is being explored. This narrative may take a number of forms depending largely upon the individual's preference. For example, a written account or a recording may be used. This will usually encompass a summary of the experience as well as an account of the personal feelings and emotions that were engendered both during and after it took place. This exercise enables the individual to 'reach back' into their memory of the experience/situation/incident in order to try and discover a greater depth of understanding of what went on and how they felt about it. Let's take as an example a fairly typical experience that a newly qualified RVN may encounter:

First level

Beth, a relatively inexperience RVN, arrived at work at 7.30 as she was on the early shift to find that an RTC had just arrived and the duty vet, also a relatively newly qualified colleague called Alison, with whom Beth had a good working relationship, was in the midst of dealing with two distraught owners and a collapsed Cockerpoo called Freddie.

Beth was aware that she had to prepare and open up the practice but was equally aware that this was an emergency and so she immediately offered her help to Alison. Beth had qualified 13 months ago and had gained a lot of routine nursing experience as well as some critical care nursing but she still felt nervous about taking the nursing lead in an emergency. Alison had joined the practice 6 months ago following graduation and this was the first serious RTC where she had sole charge. Beth offered to take the owners into the client's quiet room whilst Alison finished her initial assessment and started treatment before moving the dog to the prep room to begin intensive support.

Beth was unable to get back to Alison as quickly as she would have liked as the owners were understandably upset and needed reassurance. She told them that she was sure that Freddie would be fine and left the room to assist Alison. When she entered the consulting room, it was apparent that Freddie had deteriorated and Alison was very stressed, as she had been trying to place a catheter unsuccessfully and looked very strained. She asked why Beth had taken so long as she had needed her help to place the catheter! Beth apologised and suggested that they take Freddie to the Prep Room immediately.

Once there they set to work placing Freddie on oxygen, setting up I.V. access and administering drugs as well as monitoring his parameters. He seemed to rally but after 15 minutes, suddenly crashed and could not be revived.

Both Alison and Beth were extremely upset, Alison because having sole responsibility for a situation of this type was a new experience for her and Beth was equally upset because she had known Freddie and his owners for some time as clients in the practice and knew them to be very caring owners of a lovely, friendly dog who was now no more.

Alison went to break the news to Freddie's owners whilst Beth started clearing up and arranging Freddie on a blanket in case his owners wanted to say goodbye.

Alison came back after 10 minutes with the owners who were distraught and when they saw her the husband said that when she (Beth) had told them that Freddie was going to be OK – she had given them some hope but that it was not to be. His tone was accusatory which compounded Beth's feelings of guilt and inadequacy.

Beth gave her condolences and left them to say goodbye to Freddie. She went into the reception area to start the process of opening the practice to find that the

Practice Manager was already there, it was apparent from his demeanour that he was unhappy that the front door was still locked and that there was a client waiting outside. Beth apologised and tried to explain but he suggested that her time would be better spent letting the client into the waiting room.

Beth carried on with her work and eventually caught up but at coffee break she broke down in tears when her best friend asked why she was so quiet. . .

Superficial reflection	Beth is competent within her sphere of experience but is still not comfortable dealing with novel situations, especially those that are 'high risk'. She possesses a degree of confidence which enables her to react with some self-possession and to carry out instruction competently.

However, she is likely to have an instinctive reaction when placed in such a novel high-stress situation – hence her suggestion to the owners that 'Freddie will be fine', which was an emotional reaction to their distress as well as a subconscious hope.

Her distress both at the death of Freddie and later on that morning will have arisen because of her sense that she had made a number of mistakes, falsely reassuring the owners, taking too long to get back to support Alison, failing to fulfil her responsibilities to open up as the 'early nurse' in the practice. These compounded a sense that she has been tested as a veterinary nurse and has failed, with the result that Freddie could not be saved. |
| Second level | Although Beth may not want to dwell on the experience whilst it is fresh in her mind, she may be helped to do so by her colleague and close friend, who may help Beth to talk through and rationalise both the situation and her emotions. Their discussion might follow these lines: |

- Beth was not the instigator of the set of circumstances that led to Freddie being involved in the accident and then being presented at the practice.
- Her action in trying to reassure the owners was well meant but misplaced, and it is one that she will not repeat in the future, having learned from this experience.
- The owners may have subconsciously looked to place some of the blame for Freddie's death on Beth's shoulders because they themselves felt a significant burden of guilt and are even now trying to rationalise their loss and asking what they could/should have done to prevent the accident.
- Alison felt out of her depth due to her inexperience and was looking for a degree of assurance from Beth, which she was unable to receive because of Beth's absence at a critical time. This was not Beth's fault as she was needed elsewhere and made a judgement to that effect. She might deal with a similar situation differently in the future, based on her increasing level of experience, Schön's Reflection-in-Action.
- The Practice Manager was focused on the smooth running of the practice and was not aware of the full extent of the emergency at the time. This gave rise to a lack of sympathy for Beth and it may be that a reflective exercise may give rise to greater insight.

Third level	A deeper level of insight that also includes ethical and 'political' may be gained by interrogating the thoughts gained from the first two stages. For example:

- Patient welfare
  - Was it compromised?
  - If yes, what lessons can be learned to ensure that the situation never arises again? Should the practice institute a policy of having two staff members on duty in the morning?
- Care of colleagues
  - Could inter-colleague communication have been better, and if so, how can this be improved? Is there an opportunity to reflect upon communication skills throughout the practice team? This must be a positive experience where the potential for any blame is avoided.
  - Should Alison offer support to Beth once things have settled down? After all, Alison will also be very upset and they have always had a good working relationship in the past, so communication is the key to ensuring that this continues.
  - Is this an opportunity for the practice to review its policy on staff support?
- Care of the owners
  - They will be grieving for Freddie, so how can the practice support them and should Beth be involved in this support?
  - It is important that proper consideration be given to the level of grief that they are experiencing, so recognition of this will be important for the clients; additionally, they may benefit from bereavement counselling.
- Care of Beth
  - In the past an experience such as the one outlined above would have been viewed as a rite of passage that would have weeded out the 'weak' from those who could 'hack it!' Nowadays there is a far greater understanding of the need to support those who are finding life difficult and that this situation is all too human and not a sign of weakness! Institutions such as the RCVS have developed programmes such as 'Mind Matters' to provide dedicated support for veterinary staff who are struggling. Beth's practice should give consideration to how it formally supports its staff whilst they are working in what is an increasingly stressful environment. Reflection can be a powerful tool that can be employed to aid in this process.

This example serves to demonstrate how a reflective approach can provide greater insight and understanding of experiences and thus opens the door to a more informed approach to future practice. Whilst this example describes a highly emotional set of circumstances, the same technique can be used to delve more deeply into any new learning experience.

The previous section serves to demonstrate that there are a significant number of approaches that can be used to aid reflection. It can be seen that they tend to fall into two main categories. First, a cyclical activity where each phase informs the next in a predictive manner and thus forms the basis for future learning. This cycle can be repeated a number of times in a spiral manner. Alternatively, a hierarchy may be implemented that asks sequential questions based upon the reflector's response to the experience or set of circumstances. There is a general consensus that the approach to reflection changes as the reflector moves from novice to experienced practitioner and gains greater inherent flexibility and insight, as originally espoused by Schön, whose reflection on/in practice theory is one of the cornerstones of reflective practice.

Many of these theories would appear to have common themes. Whereas Schön describes a different philosophical approach to reflective technique in the experienced as opposed to the inexperienced practitioner, others such as Kolb, Goodman, John, and Levee use the aforementioned cyclical or building block approach where the ability to reflect, both on individual events and as a reflective practitioner in general, is enhanced by revisiting the process one or more times, and at each visit being able to learn from the change in perspective.

In some respects, this is to be expected in that the more a skill or cognitive task is repeated, the more accomplished the individual will become. However, there is also a philosophical element to consider in that reflection is primarily an exercise in developing self-awareness and using this to enhance the individual's interaction with the external environment. This requires guidance in order that the new perspective can be measured against what is considered normal or correct. For example, clinical competence in taking a blood sample is reliant upon the correct procedure being demonstrated to the student in the first place. The student can then reflect on their own experience of performing the skill to facilitate an improvement in practice. However, it would be difficult to engage in a reflective approach from the outset without the guidelines to work with. Mantzoukas (2007) discusses the concept of students creating their own understanding of knowledge by means of a reflective epistemology, which facilitates a learning environment where the teacher becomes another enquirer with a similar status to the students. In the past this would not have sat well in the didactic world of formal education and would have been resisted by many teachers/lecturers, who favoured a teacher- rather than student-centred approach. However, it has significant merit within veterinary practice where a team-based and in many cases a problem-based learning (PBL) approach is more readily adopted. This has considerable merit in the training environment as the clinical coach/mentor and the student are able to work towards set objectives as a team.

Application in the Classroom and Workplace

The early days of UK veterinary nurse training mirrored that of the State Registered Nurse (SRN) qualification in medicine. The teaching of practical skills was at its core and students spent most of their training in the workplace. This allowed them to engage and become familiar with the reality of nursing whilst learning on the job, but it did not facilitate reflection. The introduction of degree-level courses at the turn of the century was something of a catalyst as it encompassed a reflective stance as part of the curriculum. It could be argued that reflective practice in general was developed, in part, as a response to the need to understand how leaning could be enhanced in the context of *reflexion*, hence the application to the working environment within the professions. This promoted the realisation that the skill could be adopted at undergraduate level and then carried into the working environment with an end result of promoting lifelong learning and CPD. In addition, it is viewed as beneficial, not only as a positive attribute for students but also a means to ensure that graduates are fit for employment.

Jack Mezirow (1990) described the significant factors in learning from practice when he discussed the issue of 'perspective transformation'. This refers to the way in which individuals gain an understanding of how and why assumptions about the world around us can constrain our perspective of ourselves and our relationships.

Mezirow described two approaches to achieving perspective transformation:

A *'light bulb moment'* which changes the way we see ourselves or the world. For example, the realisation that we hold a particular belief system that influences our response to a client's circumstances.

Critical reflectivity – perspective transformation is achieved by proceeding though a series of small modifications where previously held assumptions are revised until they are transformed. Mezirow identified six stages, or levels, of reflectivity:

Level	Definition	Questions which may be used in a critical incident event
Reflectivity	The ability to observe and describe – being aware of the surroundings	Describe the experience, what did I observe?
Affective reflectivity	Internal awareness – our thoughts feelings and actions	What were my initial thoughts during and immediately after the incident? How did I feel during and afterwards?
Discriminant reflectivity	Knowledge of how circumstances influence the process of decision-making	What factors made me act/respond in the manner that I did? Do I need to alter this and if so how?
Judgemental reflectivity	Awareness of our own values and assumptions and their effect on our decision-making	Agyris – (see earlier) described the individual's mind map of probable experience outcomes based on previous experience and underpinning knowledge. This will also be influenced by an individual's cultural background and assumptions.
Conceptual reflectivity	Knowledge of the underlying concepts and how they are used in clinical decision-making. This includes the ability to know when there are gaps in our knowledge	The experienced reflective practitioner will not be afraid of challenging themselves and their own practice with a view to altering their perspective if necessary.
Theoretical reflectivity	The influence of formal theory and underpinning knowledge on clinical practice as well as the effect that pre-existing experience combines with this to influence perceptions and actions	Whilst the experienced practitioner will take a flexible approach to the need to change their practice if necessary, the novice will be more reliant on the theoretical knowledge

(From Mezirow 1990).

The publication of the Dearing Report in 1997, and its subsequent endorsement by the UK Government, facilitated a significant change in the delivery of higher education in the UK. One important element of the Report was the recommendation that the process of student education should be enriched by means of the introduction of a more reflective approach to learning. It was envisaged that this would be facilitated by use of individual student Progress Files (PF) that would enable each student to record their academic progress, including the gaining of transferable skills and personal development, and it would also encourage them to engage in deeper learning by means of the reflective process required to undertake *Personal* Development Planning (PDP).

Reflective practice is a transferable skill and as such its use has been adopted in higher education as an integral element of a continuum of learning that extends beyond graduation into the workplace. This fits with the concept of lifelong learning as described earlier. However, it is essential that not only should professional or vocational competence be documented, but also that the individual's ability to reflect upon the learning experience is facilitated. This has led to the implementation of a variety of methods of documenting such evidence, including reflective diaries and computer-based packages that allow students to record their achievement, the most useful of which can be accessed via a smartphone, which makes the record both flexible and portable.

The RCVS requirement for recording CPD is facilitated by means of an online program, the most recent iteration being 1 CPD. The present requirement for Registered Veterinary Nurses is 15 hours CPD per year, with the requirement for the documentation of reflection on the activity. Equally, student veterinary nurses are encouraged to automatically engage in reflection as part of their learning and assessment, thus developing the mindset for their future career once qualified.

This concept of staff-facilitated but student-driven reflection was advocated by Dearing as a way of enabling students to identify personal and academic weak areas. It can also be viewed as a tool that will increase graduate employability by means of developing the skills and attributes that are valued by employers, such as the ability to communicate well and high levels of motivation.

Focus must be on supporting students to understand the theory of reflective practice and how it can be implemented to improve theoretical engagement and practical skills. In addition, the other significant objective that must be achieved is sustained and effective engagement between the formal teaching institution and the satellite veterinary practices that facilitate the all-important student placements. The goal should be the development of a supportive community that combines theoretical and skills-based learning with the individual student's needs at the centre of that provision.

Teaching and Mentoring Reflective Practice

Extensive consideration as evidenced in the supportive learning texts demonstrates that the process of reflection is now more readily accepted by professional programmes such as nursing and teaching, where the ability to learn from the vocational experience has been a critical part of student development for some time.

Clegg and Bradley (2006) conducted 32 semi-structured interviews over a nine-week period in 2002/2003 to ascertain staff acceptance of PDP. Reponses appeared to indicate that the implementation of the process was largely unsuccessful for a variety of reasons. These included the fact that systems were introduced without sufficient explanation to staff and students alike. They concluded that there would appear to be considerable evidence that some staff felt that they did not have the skills to support reflection and that the same individuals also questioned its usefulness among groups of students who were not predisposed to engage.

The reality for many staff members is that they even if they are so inclined, they do not have the luxury of sufficient time available to devote to the development of the process and to its implementation. So, what can be done to make this process easier? The cornerstones of reflective facilitation are:

- Early adoption and familiarisation with the concept by the student.
- Selection of suitable staff members within the workplace who are happy to engage in the process and support students. Once in the role they should receive suitable training to accomplish this role as well as regular protected time to support their students
- Recognition by the veterinary team that the ability to reflect is a transferable skill that enhances nursing skills and patient welfare, and as such should be embedded in the Clinical Coach/Mentor role, which should be fully recognised as being part of career progression. The addition of a degree of financial reward within the organisation's salary structure would add to its perceived status.
- The development of the ethos of integral reflection as part of day-to-day practice so that it becomes second nature. This starts with the student, who will then instil it into their students as they progress along their career path and become experts in their own right.

Taking Benner's continuum as a template, it can be seen that that, whilst the student nurse has the greatest requirement for teaching and support within the veterinary practice, learning, and by default teaching, does not cease upon qualification. Rather it should be an activity that continues throughout the whole of an individual's career, as there is always something new to learn. The engagement with reflection helps to enhance this as it opens the mind to possibilities that an individual may not have been aware of previously. In addition, there is a place for the support of less experienced staff members by those with greater skill and experience, such as may be found in the preceptor relationship. Also known in some spheres as clinical trainers, preceptors provide support for their junior colleagues over a set period of time governed by discrete goals such as working towards a post entry-level qualification or in order to gain further experience within a particular discipline. The use of a reflective learning approach between colleagues in this context allows for an enhanced experience, which can be beneficial for both parties.

The mentor/clinical coach will often be the staff member who facilitates reflection for the student, and the role carries a significant level of responsibility. They should ideally have a number of attributes including the ability to engender trust and possess good listening skills. Regular opportunities for discussion and feedback will allow for feedback and identification of a particular focus for reflection as training progresses.

Conclusion

Reflection is now perceived to be an integral part of the initial learning process and subsequent professional development in nursing. As such, it is expected that both institutions as well as regulatory professional bodies will embed reflective skills teaching and support into their curricula and CPD guidance to facilitate this element of learning and professional practice. Critics may submit that there is a slavish adoption to the philosophy and that whilst it easy to teach the concepts, it is harder for some individuals to embrace the skill and as such this can act as a barrier. In addition, constant questioning can lead to stasis if it results in the undermining of confidence, leading to an inability to progress. However, nowadays the general consensus is that reflection enriches the learning process and enables the expert and novice alike to make sense of their working environment, which engenders greater flexibility.

Whilst it is undoubtedly easier for some than for others to embrace reflective practice, the embedding of a reflective ethos is now accepted as an essential element of informed practice within the professions. In veterinary nursing, it can serve to enhance best practice and improve animal welfare and, in addition, it develops a personal insight that can enrich the individual's self-worth. It does come with inherent risks as self-awareness can lead to an undermining of personal confidence if managed badly, and for this reason the tutor/clinical coach plays a critical role in managing a supportive reflective environment and should be provided with the tools and the time to deliver this important function.

References

Agyris, C. and Schon, D.A. (1974). *Theory in Practice: Increasing Professional Effectiveness.* San Francisco, CA: Jossey-Bass.

Benner, P. (1984). *From Novice to Expert.* Menlo Park, CA: Addison–Wesley.

Borton, T. (1970). *Reach, Touch and Teach.* London: Hutchinson.

Boud, D., Keogh, R., and Walker, D. (1985). *Reflection: Turning Experience into Learning.* London: Kogan Page Ltd.

Brockbank, A. and McGill, I. (1998). *Facilitating Reflective Learning in Higher Education.* Buckingham: Society for Research into Higher Education and Open University Press.

Brookfield, S. (1993). Self-directed learning, political clarity, and the critical practice of adult education. *Adult Educ. Q.* 43 (4): 227–242.

Caldwell, L. and Grobbel, C.C. (2013). The importance of reflective practice in nursing. *Int. J. Caring Sci.* 6 (3): 319–326.

Carper, B. (1978). Fundamental patterns of knowing in nursing. *Adv. Nurs. Sci.* 1 (1): 13–23.

Collins English Dictionary (1988). *Chambers English Dictionary*. Cambridge: Cambridge University Press.

Clegg, S. (2004). Critical readings: progress files and the production of the autonomous learner. *Teach. High. Educ.* 9 (3): 287–298.

Clegg, S. and Bradley, S. (2006). The implementation of progress files in higher education: reflection as national policy. *High. Educ.* 51: 465–486.

Dearing, R. (1997). *Higher Education in the Learning Society*. Norwich: HMSO.

Dewey, J. (1933). *A Restatement of the Relation of Reflective Thinking to the Educative Process*. Boston, MA: D.C. Heath & Co. Publishers.

Gibbs, G. (1988). *Learning by Doing: A Guide to Teaching and Learning Methods*. Oxford: Oxford Brooks University.

Goodman, J. (1984). Reflection and teacher education: a case study ad theoretic analysis. *Interchange* 15 (3): 9–26.

Honey, P. and Mumford, A. (1992). *The Manual of Learning Styles*. Maidenhead: Peter Honey.

Jasper, M. (2003). *Beginning Reflective Practice*. Cheltenham: Nelson Thornes Ltd.

Johns, C. (1995). Framing learning through reflection within carpers fundamental ways of knowing in nursing. *J. Adv. Nurs.* 22: 226–234.

Jootun, D. and McGarry, W. (2014). Reflection in nurse education. *J. Nurs. Care* 3 (2): 148–150.

Kolb, D.A. (1984). *Experiential Leaning: Experience as the Source of Learning and Development*. Englewood Cliffs, NJ: Prentice-Hall.

Larrivee, B. (2008). Development of a tool to assess teacher's reflective practice. *Reflective Pract* 9: 341–360.

Mantzoukas, S. (2007). Reflection and problem/enquiry based learning: confluences and contradictions. *Reflective Pract.* 8 (2): 241–253.

Mezirow, J. (1990). *Fostering Critical Reflection in Adulthood : A Guide to Transformative and Emancipatory Learning*. San Francisco, CA: Jossey-Bass.

Schön, D.A. (1987). *Educating the Reflective Practitioner: Toward a New Design of Teaching and Learning in the Professions*. San Francisco, CA: Jossey Bass.

Stephenson, A.M. and Burns, S. (1994). *Reflective Practice in Nursing: The Growth of the Professional Practitioner*, 5e. Oxford: Wiley Blackwell.

Wallace, M. (1996). When is experiential learning not experiential learning? In: *Liberating the Learner: Lessons for Professional Development in Education* (ed. T. Atkinson, G. Claxton, M. Osborn and M. Wallace), 16–31. London: Routledge.

Further reading

Ashraf, H. and Rarieya, J. (2008). Teacher development through reflective conversations – possibilities and tensions: a Pakistan case. *Reflective Pract.* 9 (3): 269–279.

Bold, C. (2008). Peer support groups: fostering a deeper approach to learning through critical reflection on practice. *Reflective Pract.* 9 (3): 257–267.

Burns, S. and Bulman, C. (1994). *Reflective Practice in Nursing*. Oxford: Blackwell Publishing.

Clegg, S., Tan, J., and Saeidi, S. (2002). Reflecting or acting? Reflective practice and continuing professional development in higher education. *Reflective Pract.* 3 (1): 132–146.

Cotton, A.H. (2001). Private thoughts in public spheres: issues in reflection and reflective practices in nursing. *J. Adv. Nurs.* 364: 512–519.

Cross, V., Liles, C., Conduit, J. et al. (2004). Linking reflective practice to evidence of competence: a workshop for allied health professional. *Reflective Pract.* 5 (1): 3–31.

Epstein, R.M. (1999). Mindful practice. *J. Am. Med. Assoc.* 282 (9): 833–839.

Fowler, J. and Chevannes, M. (1998). Evaluating the efficacy of reflective practice within the context of clinical supervision. *J. Adv. Nurs.* 27: 379–382.

Ghaye, T. (2007). Is reflective practice ethical? *Reflective Pract.* 8 (2): 151–162.

Ghaye, T. and Lillyman, S. (2000). *Reflection: Principles and Practice for Healthcare Professionals*. Dinton: Quay Books.

Glaze, J.E. (2001). Reflection as a transforming process: student advanced nurse practitioners' experiences of developing reflective skills as part of an MSc programme. *J. Adv. Nurs.* 345: 639–647.

Glaze, J.E. (2002). Stages in coming to terms with reflection: student advanced nurse Practitioners' perceptions of their reflective journeys. *J. Adv. Nurs.* 373: 265–272.

Haigh, J. (2008). Integrating progress files in the academic process: a review of case studies. *Act. Learn. High. Educ.* 9 (1): 57–71.

Hannigan, B. (2001). A discussion of the strengths and weaknesses of 'reflection' in nursing practice and education. *J. Clin. Nurs.* 102: 278–283.

Hillier, Y. (2002). *Reflective Teaching in Further and Adult Education*. London: Continuum.

Johns, C. (1994). Nuances of reflection. *J. Clin. Nurs.* (3, 2): 71–74.

Johns, C. (2000). *Becoming a Reflective Practitioner: A Reflective and Holistic Approach to Clinical Nursing, Practice Development and Clinical Supervision*. Oxford: Blackwell Science.

Johns, C. and Freshwater, D. (ed.) (1998). *Transforming Nursing through Reflective Practice*. Oxford: Blackwell Science.

Longenecker, R. (2002). The jotter wallet: invoking reflective practice in a family practice residency program. *Reflective Pract.* 3 (2): 219–224.

Maich, N.M., Brown, B., and Royle, J. (2000). 'Becoming' through reflection and professional portfolios: the voice of growth in nurses. *Reflective Pract.* 1 (3): 309–324.

Miller, A. (2005). Reflection on the preparation and implementation of a practicum designed for a junior physiotherapist in primary care. *Reflective Pract.* 6 (1): 15–32.

Moon, J.A. (1999). *Reflection in Learning & Professional Development: Theory & Practice*. London: Kogan Page Ltd.

Mountford, B. and Rogers, L. (1996). Assessing individual and group reflection in and on assessment as a tool for effective learning. *J. Adv. Nurs.* 24: 1127–1134.

Myrick, F. and Yonge, O.J. (2001). Creating a climate for critical thinking in the preceptorship experience. *Nurse Educ. Today* 21: 461–467.

Newton, J.M. (2000). Uncovering knowing in practice amongst a group of undergraduate student nurses. *Reflective Pract.* 1 (2): 184–197.

Nikolou-Walker, E. and Garnett, J. (2004). Work-based learning. A new imperative: developing reflective practice in professional life. *Reflective Pract.* 5 (3): 297–312.

O'Connor, A., Hyde, A., and Treacy, M.P. (2003). Nurse teacher's constructions of reflection and reflective practice. *Reflective Pract.* 4 (2): 108–119.

Osterman, K.F. and Kottkamp, R.B. (1993). *Reflective Practice for Educators: Improving Schooling through Professional Development*. Thousand Oaks, CA: Corwin Press Inc.

Ottesen, E. (2007). Reflection in teacher education. *Reflective Pract.* 8 (1): 31–46.

Pierson, W. (1998). Reflection and nursing education. *J. Adv. Nurs.* 27: 165–170.

Raw, J., Brigden, D., and Gupta, R. (2005). Reflective diaries in medical practice. *Reflective Pract.* 6 (1): 165–169.

Rees, C.E., Shepherd, M., and Chamberlain, S. (2005). The utility of reflective portfolios as a method of assessing first year medical students' personal and professional development. *Reflective Pract.* 6 (1): 3–14.

Regan, P. (2008). Reflective practice: how far how deep? *Reflective Pract.* 9 (2): 219–229.

Russell, T. (2005). Can reflective practice be taught? *Reflective Pract.* 6 (2): 199–204.

Scanlan, J.M., Care, W.D., and Udod, S. (2002). Unravelling the unknowns of reflection in classroom teaching. *J. Adv. Nurs.* 382: 136–143.

Sparrow, J., Ashford, R., and Heel, D. (2005). A methodology to identify workplace features that can facilitate or impede reflective practice: a national health service UK study. *Reflective Pract.* 6 (2): 190–196.

Taylor, B.J. (2000). *Reflective Practice: A Guide for Nurses and Midwives*. Buckingham: Open University.

Thorpe, K. (2004). Reflective learning journals: from concept to practice. *Reflective Pract.* 5 (3): 328–343.

Upton, D. and Upton, P. (2006). Development of an evidence-based practice questionnaire for nurses. *J. Adv. Nurs.* 54 (4): 454–458.

Watson, J.S. and Wilcox, S. (2000). Reading for understanding: methods of reflecting on practice. *Reflective Pract.* 1 (1): 57–67.

9 The RVN's Role in Evidence-Based Veterinary Nursing

Sarah Batt-Williams and Lyndsay Wade

What Is Evidence-Based Veterinary Nursing and Why Should Veterinary Nurses Be Involved?

Evidence-Based Veterinary Nursing (EBVN), also known as Evidence-Based Veterinary Medicine (EBVM) depending on the topic, is the way in which the profession will develop and ultimately the care that is provided to patients will improve. This may arise via enhancements in customer relations, inter-team communications, practice policies, or One Health or nursing interventions. EBVN is the combination of using the best available evidence, professional expertise and opinion, and the patient's and client's values and needs to decide on the best course of action for a patient, as shown in Figure 9.1.

By having a structured approach to the care delivered, nurses can justify the decisions made and have confidence in the rationale behind why tasks are completed in that manner. It allows the practitioner to question past practice and make robust clinical decisions, based on results from studies that are clinically relevant to the setting, rather than solely on experience, or just the client's wishes, which may not be best practice. However, EBVN does not discount these factors, it is the combination of all three which is where its strengths lie.

In order to work in an evidence-based manner, evidence must always be sought. However, it does not end there; the outcomes following the use of the evidence base in practice must also be analysed and the cycle completed with data collection by the individual. This chapter aims to explore the combination of searching the existing evidence base and the contribution made to it by veterinary nurses.

Practical Use of Evidence in the Veterinary Practice

Consider the following hypothetical scenario and evidence base. The practice you work in has a standard operating procedure (SOP), that all patients who have undergone orthopaedic surgery are hospitalised for six days postoperatively so that

Professionalism and Reflection in Veterinary Nursing, First Edition.
Edited by Sue Badger and Andrea Jeffery.
© 2022 John Wiley & Sons Ltd. Published 2022 by John Wiley & Sons Ltd.
Companion website: www.wiley.com/go/badger/professionalism-veterinary-nursing

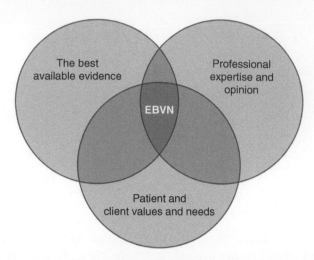

Figure 9.1 Contributory factors for EBVN. Source: Adapted from Studer and Abbott (2020).

they can receive two days of methadone, two days of buprenorphine, and then two days of oral medications before being discharged. You are admitting a patient who will undergo this process and the owner expresses concern about being away from their family member for so long. They question why it must be at least six days and you reply that it is practice policy. However, this makes you think about whether this is best practice. You ask the team and there are varying opinions, some had never thought to question the practice protocol, but the general consensus is that a patient requires six days of intravenous analgesia before mobilising comfortably. You decide to review the evidence base and find that studies reported the use of a validated pain scale allowed the analgesia doses, frequency, and duration to be tailored to the patient, often resulting in shorter hospitalisation durations. You present this to the veterinary team for a discussion, and it is decided that this process will be followed for this patient and that a change to the SOP will be considered. You therefore inform the owner that whilst the length of stay may not change, the patient will only be hospitalised for the duration required.

In this scenario the evidence base has allowed the tradition of the six-day postoperative care to be tailored to the patient and owner's needs, whilst harnessing the best practice possible. If the veterinary nurse were to be questioned as to the decision-making behind this strategy, there would be a systematic approach to the care provided. The veterinary nurse who conducted the literature search may then wish to collate their findings and publish this information in the form of a literature review or a critically appraised topic such as a Knowledge Summary (RCVS Knowledge 2021a) or BestBET for Vets (University of Nottingham 2021) so that others with the same question can access the information. Furthermore, the nurse and veterinary team should document their experiences of the change in protocol, ensuring that the change has been positive and there is an improvement in the care provided to the patient and the service provided to the client. This data collection may again be published to enhance the existing evidence base.

Benefits of Evidence-Based Veterinary Nursing and Research for the Individual

Whilst the introduction to this chapter has explored why *veterinary nurses* should undertake EBVN, it is also important to explore the benefits for the individual. Why should *you* be interested in this topic? Practice-based veterinary nurses are in a unique position to identify problems and/or areas for improvements in the quality of veterinary care. This is also true in the medical (human-centred) nursing profession, as clinical nurses often become research-active when driven by a clinical trigger (Siedlecki and Albert 2017). By investigating the questions that you have in the practice, you will be able to think critically about the decisions you make and justify your nursing practices. Not only does this offer you the confidence to implement the best patient and client care, it can also provide enhanced job satisfaction (Hauser and Jackson 2017) and greater autonomy. Furthermore, EBVN is part of clinical governance, which is incorporated in the Code of Professional Conduct for nurses and the Practice Standards Scheme (RCVS Knowledge 2021b).

Additionally, this process allows you to explore topics in greater detail and become more knowledgeable in the field of study. Being a knowledgeable person in a specific field of practice means that you may be asked to speak at conferences, write articles or book chapters, it may open job opportunities that you had never considered or mean that you are a more competitive candidate for your ideal job. Hauser and Jackson (2017) further explore the non-clinical benefits of EBVN in their open access article.

The RVN as a Clinical Researcher

Becoming a clinical researcher seems a daunting task, one that historically people may not have felt was within the role of the veterinary nurse. A traditional view of research is a person in a lab wearing a white coat and goggles or working in academia studying complex or rare diseases. Whilst in some circumstances, this is what a researcher is, the clinical researchers in this chapter are veterinary nurses working in the veterinary practice with patients, their owners, and the veterinary team, searching for answers to common clinical questions.

RCVS Knowledge detail five steps to EBVN and in undertaking this process, the veterinary nurse becomes a clinical researcher as these are the first steps of research:

1. Convert information needs into answerable questions.
2. Track down the best evidence with which to answer them.
3. Critically appraise the evidence for validity.
4. Apply the results to clinical practice.
5. Evaluate performance.

(RCVS Knowledge 2021c)

A lack of existing evidence within veterinary nursing, however, may mean that reaching the latter steps of the five-step approach is challenging and therefore balancing the three components of evidence-based practice becomes impossible. The lack of evidence base within the profession becomes a negative feedback loop. Without an evidence base, the profession cannot work in an evidence-based manner, there is then a lack of role models and examples of evidence-based practice to follow. Only members of the profession can put an end to this cycle through contributions to the evidence base. Figure 9.2 demonstrates the steps a nurse would take if they were to find a lack of evidence base.

Do Veterinary Nurses Have the Correct Skills and Training to Undertake EBVN and Data Collection?

Suggesting that the profession should address this issue and begin to research would rely on its members having the appropriate skills and training to do so. No matter which route of training is taken, an RVN will have the required level of Maths, English, and analytical skills to be involved in reviewing the evidence base and applying the information. This is the foundation of the first two parts of this chapter.

The remainder of the chapter will consider how data may be collected to answer a clinical question. This will focus on the introduction of *quantitative research* as, again, RVNs have the skills required to collect data from their pre-registration training but may just need to learn the process. *Qualitative research*, however, requires greater understanding of human interaction and social research *methods*, which is beyond the scope of this chapter to explore. Therefore, specialist resources should be utilised for the later sections of this chapter if you are considering a qualitative study.

Considering undertaking research may, again, seem daunting. However, another fundamental aspect of veterinary nursing is teamwork, which is essential in EBVN. Whilst a veterinary nurse can work individually on a topic, working in a team is always beneficial to spread the workload and increase the diversity of ideas. Furthermore, starting on an evidence-based journey with a mentor in research, or a specialist in the subject that you are initially exploring, can be incredibly valuable for confidence and guidance. This mentor may be a person within your practice or chain, a former colleague, or a peer. You may even wish to email a local college or university who may have someone that would be able to provide support. The latter would be mutually beneficial, as those working in such roles often have requirements to be involved in research. Likewise, for those outside of academia, the individual benefits of contributing to EBVN will still apply to the mentor. Finally, there are many post-registration veterinary nursing courses that could be undertaken if this chapter inspires you but does not provide you with the full confidence or understanding to go it alone!

Final Thoughts

You may have identified with some of the topics raised so far and have been persuaded to begin to investigate the research journey further. This chapter will explore the first steps to becoming a clinical researcher, what processes you would

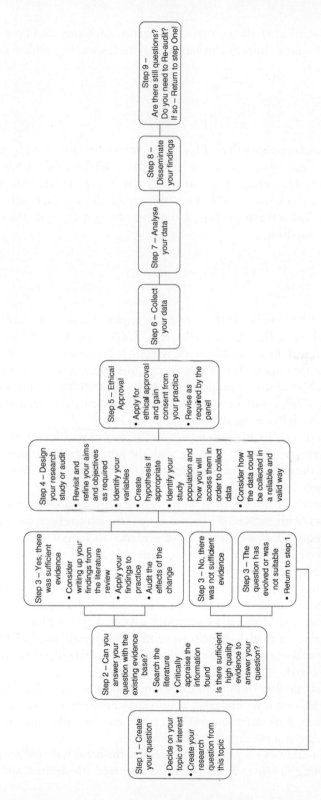

Figure 9.2 Designing and implementing a research study.

be likely to follow, what challenges you may face at each step and how those may be overcome and where support can be gained, from sourcing evidence to collecting your own data.

Critical Analysis and Asking the Research Question

The initial step when working in an EBVN manner, as demonstrated by both RCVS Knowledge and Figure 9.2, is to create a question. Whilst this sounds simplistic, creating an answerable, achievable, and relevant question is often one of the most time-consuming aspects of EBVN. This section of the chapter will guide you through the question writing process; from identifying a topic to the creation of a robust clinical question.

The Research Topic

All research must be beneficial; there must be a purpose in its outcome in order to justify its existence. Therefore, whilst the EBVN topic must be of interest to you, the clinical researcher, it must also be worthwhile to conduct and have benefits to the project's *stakeholders*. When considering the topic, a natural place to start, as *reflective practitioners*, is reflection. The tasks that veterinary nurses complete daily within their roles will have an impact on patient, clients, the team, and themselves and can initiate the reflective process.

As an example, take a moment to reflect on the way in which you clean a kennel. For most nurses this will involve starting with the area of least contact (the ceiling) moving towards the area of greatest potential contamination (the floor and bars). Indeed, this seems logical, or perhaps it is not something that you have ever considered. However, if the cleaning agent can destroy organisms in the presence of organic matter with sufficient contact time, you may reflect on whether this method is still required. If we do not have evidence to support this method, then we are simply hoping that logic is correct. A decade ago, it was common practice to scruff cats and restrain them in a full body hold, yet research has demonstrated that this is a noxious experience (Moody et al. 2018) and now it is something that has been banned in most practices. Cleaning a kennel in the top to bottom approach is as widely accepted as scruffing cats was, yet within the veterinary sector, it is not known if it does help to reduce pathogenic loads. EBVN allows these sorts of clinical questions to be posed and then answered, stimulating further questions to be asked.

Whilst the vast number of clinical questions will arise from daily tasks, topics of interest may also become apparent following unexpected events such as feedback from a client, a negative outcome in a patient, or following conversations with colleagues about a recently published article.

Frameworks of analysis may be used to identify the areas where there are clinical questions remaining or where an incident has occurred which the team would like to address. Structure may be provided by reflective models such as Kolb (1984) and Gibbs' (1988) or critical incident analysis models such as *Root Cause Analysis* (RCVS Knowledge 2020a).

You may wish to complete Exercise 9.1, to review which questions may be beneficial to ask in your practice.

Approaches to Finding the Research Question

Once a broad topic has been identified, the clinical researcher can begin to consider their approach to the question. It may be that a question within a topic has been identified that they would like to explore further, by collecting data to construct a theory; this is an inductive approach. Alternatively, the clinical researcher may have a theory or observation that has been noticed, which then becomes the focus of the project and is tested; this is a deductive approach. As an example, the research topic may ask which tape is the most suitable to secure intravenous catheters. With an inductive approach the question may be which catheter tape would be best by comparing two commonly used varieties. With a deductive approach, it may have already been noticed that one tape has superior qualities and so the two tapes in the practice are tested to see if there was valid evidence behind the observation.

Once a topic and an approach are identified, the clinical researcher should consider what it is that they would like to find out specifically and if it will be of benefit to spend time and resources to find this out. Not only does this ensure that the project will be worthwhile, it also aids the researcher in the construction of an appropriate question.

Complete Exercise 9.2 to highlight this further.

Refining the Research Question

The research question is fundamental to the whole EBVN process. Every subsequent step relies on an appropriate question; therefore, it is of upmost importance that the greatest amount of time and consideration is paid to it. A research question defines the topic of study, provides it with a clear purpose, influences the research design and allows visualisation of the outcomes. This is the same whether you are creating a research question upon which to conduct a literature search or you have completed a literature search and now wish to undertake a clinical study.

A good clinical research question is one that is answerable. This may sound simplistic; however, it takes time, consideration, and many edits to ensure a research question can be answered. Once the broad topic has been narrowed to a single question, it should be considered what each of the key themes in the question means so that the researcher can refine the question further and fully understand the scope of the literature search and any subsequent data collection.

For example, the earlier example question, 'Which is the most suitable catheter tape to use in this practice?', may be broken down as follows:

- *Which:* There will be some form of comparison of which tape is used in practice, is this inductive or deductive?
- *Most suitable:* This suggests that there will be superior qualities of one over another, what are these qualities?
- *Catheter tape:* What constitutes catheter tape? How many options are available? Will the tape only be considered for this use?
- *To use:* Will this become a practice protocol – will the research be able to answer this as will it vary from practice to practice based on availability, price, and patient factors?
- *In this practice:* Is this all patients in the practice? Can this be generalised to other practices, for example within the group or chain?

Once all parts of the question are considered you should have a better understanding of what it is that you are trying to find out.

From this exercise, it is evident that there are many additional questions within the question and it therefore requires further editing to ensure that it is answerable and achievable. This is where three mnemonics can be used to structure the question further, these are SMART, PICO, and FINER.

The SMART mnemonic acronym originally developed by Doran (1981) for objective setting, can be adapted to define and refine the research question to make it answerable. The letters spell out specific, measurable, achievable, realistic, and timely.

- Specific – The question must be precise about what it is the researcher is trying to find out, identifying a clear outcome.
- Measurable – The outcome should be quantifiable, meaning that the topic can be physically measured by collecting information or data to produce results.
- Achievable and Realistic – There must be a way to find out the answer and it must be within the researcher's access to resources to find out.
- Timely – How long can the researcher devote to finding this answer out and is the data that the question relates to influenced by time?

When applying this back to the catheter tape scenario, each of the themes within the question needs to be specified. The clinical researcher is interested in which tape is the most suitable to use for securing intravenous catheters, however, what does most suitable mean? 'Most suitable' could mean different things to different people. For example, most suitable for the practice manager may mean cheapest, for the patient, the most comfortable, and for the nurse, the most secure. If you tried to consider all three at once it would be challenging to compare these factors, for example, if it was found that tape 1 caused the least skin irritation but cost more than the practice could afford, the research is not useful at the point that it is required, the veterinary practice, so again what is 'most suitable?' The question needs refining further, perhaps the overarching consideration for the clinical researcher is a reduction in complications. Once the research is complete, whether that is a literature review or whether enough evidence and data was collected by the practice, the practice may then rank the tapes in order of fewest number of complications to greatest and then purchase the highest ranked tape that they can afford. Applying this to the question, it would change to, 'Does tape 1, 2, or 3 cause the fewest complications when securing intravenous catheters?'. The researcher could define what they meant by complications, for example dislodgment, patient interference, and skin irritation. This would not need to appear in the question, but the researcher would need to define this for themself, as for example if the researcher found 10 studies to answer their question, but all compared different complications, it would again be difficult to compare one set of results with another.

This is, however, still a challenging question to answer as the study population is vast and varied, for example, there may be species, breed, and age variations within the question. It could take years to collate enough clinical data, whether that is reviewing the evidence or undertaking the study, to be able to answer a question for all species, ages, etc. It may also not be comparable even then, and so the question, once again, is still not answerable.

Additionally, research will never provide a definitive answer; there is always some degree of variability. Therefore, to make this question SMART, it may be presented as 'Is tape 1, 2, or 3, associated with the fewest complications when securing intravenous catheters in dogs?'. This question is now specific, measurable, and achievable.

Time is considered in terms of how long the clinical researcher will spend on this project. Gannt charts are useful in organising timeframes and ordering competing time pressures. Again, this aspect does not need to come into the question; however, it is of vital importance to ensure that a nurse is using their time efficiently.

The second mnemonic which a research question should fit into is PICO. Some may find it easier to write their question in terms of SMART initially and then consider PICO, whereas others may find it easier to follow the PICO format first and then ensure it is SMART. PICO stands for:

- Patient or population: how is the population best described?
- Intervention: what is it that is being implemented in the study that you are interested in?
- Comparison: what is it that you are comparing your intervention to?
- Outcome: what are you trying to find out?

In relation to the catheter example, the PICO structure would be as depicted in Figure 9.3.

The format of PICO is flexible as, for example, in some studies there may be no comparison and the data only focuses on the outcome of an intervention. If a clinical researcher was interested in pain scales following the practice's standard pain protocol, it would be unethical to compare this to no pain relief at all; however, if the practice does not have an alternative, then there would be no

Patient or population	Dogs
Intervention	Tape 1
Comparison	Tape 2 and 3
Outcome	Fewest complications when used to secure intravenous (IV) catheters

Figure 9.3   PICO format example.

comparison in this study. The patients would therefore be scored after the intervention of the standard analgesia protocol and the researcher would then be able to ascertain whether the standard protocol provided appropriate analgesia for patients and, if not, whether additional medications could be sought.

The final mnemonic, FINER, stands for:

- Feasible – Is the question achievable and answerable? Are there funds and resources available to answer it?
- Interesting – If the research is only interesting to the clinical researcher and does not benefit the stakeholders, then it is not ethical to utilise resources to conduct it.
- Novel – If someone has already answered this question successfully, then it is again, unethical to spend resources trying to re-answer it unless the question has evolved.
- Ethical – The question must be able to be answered in an ethical manner without harming the participants.
- Relevant – The research question must be of benefit to the field of interest.

FINER will be explored further later in this chapter. It is, however, important to consider at the research question writing phase. For example, if the research question is not ethical then there will not be an evidence base to answer the question and the clinical researcher must not try to answer it themselves as this too would be unethical.

It could be argued that the research question could be even more specific, for example which vein is being utilised or in combination with which type of catheter; however, a balance must be sought between being specific enough that the question is answerable, but not so specific that the results become meaningless if applied to any other context. The topic will determine the level of specificity required and the point at which the answer will no longer be generalisable and therefore useful to add to the evidence base.

Final Thoughts

This section has explored how a clinical question may be created in terms of the original idea and how it should then be structured. The next step is to explore the literature. However, before moving on, you may wish to undertake Exercise 9.3.

Reviewing the Evidence – Conducting a Literature Review

The Importance of Reviewing the Evidence Base

Following the formulation of the research question, the clinical researcher can begin to take steps to find answers, this starts with the literature review. A logical strategy enables a thorough search and a structured process for critiquing the literature, these are required to allow the researcher to be confident in their result following a review of the evidence base.

Where to Find Evidence

To find literature, *databases* should be utilised. Databases return published literature from a specific field of interest based on the search strategy used by the author. This differs from a search engine which will return all types of information that can be found on a topic, which can be overwhelming and time-consuming to filter out what is required.

When searching literature, a range of databases should be utilised to ensure that the clinical researcher finds the best available evidence for their question. The research question and topic will determine the database utilised. For example, MEDLINE® may be utilised if it is a medical question, CINAHL® returns papers from the allied nursing professions, and similarly CAB Abstracts contains abstracts on life sciences. The benefits of these databases are that they are not linked to any one publishing group, and a thorough search may therefore be conducted. However, the research paper itself is not always found in these databases, instead a link may be provided to the publisher's database such as Science Direct for Elsevier publications. In these locations, suggested articles will often also be provided, linked to the originally searched paper, which can be beneficial. A range of databases should be accessed to prevent bias towards a single publisher, missing other publications listed elsewhere.

Google Scholar® is also commonly used and can be useful in the initial search to gauge what is known about the research question topic. However, as stated by the company itself, using this resource results in a broad range of subjects and content type, and therefore this may result in vast amounts of information, which then must be refined.

How to Search the Literature

To find information specific to your research question within a database, a search strategy is required. The key points to note are to first define the search terms, then to define the Boolean operators required, and finally to input these for the maximum effect.

To identify search terms, the key words within the research question can be highlighted and then synonyms and associated words for each word considered to aid

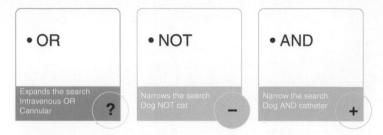

Figure 9.4   Boolean operators.

the search, as demonstrated in 'EBVM Toolkit 2: Finding the best available evidence' (RCVS Knowledge 2020b). These keywords can then be used in combination with Boolean operators to direct the search. Boolean operators, displayed in Figure 9.4, allow the expansion or refinement of the search by linking the search terms.

Once these terms have been decided, they can be inputted in the search box of the database. You may have the option to refine the search further via the advanced search function, dependening on the database and, as required, relevant to the research question.

Snowballing may also be used as a search strategy; this is the use of the reference list in the original paper that you have found to explore other papers of relevance and so on. It also includes the utilisation of the function of some databases to highlight other papers that cited the paper that you are viewing. This can flag up papers that were not in your original search but are linked. It is also time-saving. However, it should be a structured process as, without a strategy, relevant research may be missed.

A final alternative strategy would be to contact RCVS Knowledge, who are able to complete literature searches for a fee (RCVS Knowledge 2021d). This is beneficial for those who have time constraints; however, one of the benefits of conducting the literature search yourself if that you build an awareness of the topic in greater detail.

You may now wish to complete Exercise 4 to apply the information so far to your question.

Outcomes of the Literature Search

Following the literature search, there are three main outcomes:

a. A wide range of literature is found.
b. A small amount of literature is found.
c. No literature is found.

If a or b are the outcomes, then the evidence base needs to be critiqued. Following this the clinical researcher can truly decide if their question has been fully answered or not.

If the outcome is c, then the researcher must consider that either the question or search strategy was not able to elicit results and needs refining, or, there is an evidence gap in existence and data needs to be collected to answer the question.

Accessing the Articles Found

By using the appropriate search strategy, if an evidence base exists, a range of results should be obtained. It must be noted, however, that at this point a considerable challenge will be met. Outside of a university or large corporation, access to full research papers is a potential barrier as the clinical researcher may find a title and abstract from their search which they wish to explore further but cannot do so without paying a fee.

The tide is turning on this and researchers are now trying to publish in a free access manner where possible. For example, some research groups such as Vet-Compass have committed to only publish in a free access manner and other researchers may have published their data on websites such as ResearchGate when allowed. However, it is still limited, as the costs of publishing are often transferred to the submitting author.

A second option is to ask an employer if there is a budget for such access to resources, as those that are supportive of EBVN may make funds available. A Continuing Professional Development budget may also be used for accessing journals or the clinical researcher could apply for a bursary to cover costs. For example, the British Veterinary Nursing Association (BVNA) allocates bursaries, some of which may be used to cover the costs of clinical research, including the initial literature search. Finally, a clinical researcher may wish to self-fund to access the required journals.

There are also cost-effective methods of purchasing research, for example RCVS Knowledge have a library service with subscriptions to numerous veterinary journals and the ability to request interlibrary loans of research papers if required (RCVS Knowledge 2021d). A paid subscription is required; however, a single financial outlay for access to a range of veterinary journals may be more cost-efficient than paying for each article separately.

This all highlights the requirement for a strategic search, via a robust clinical question. It also means that the researcher must be reasonably confident that the evidence will be worth paying for, which is where the critical analysis of the information presented prior to paying is critical.

Critical Analysis of a Paper before Paying

When considering if it is justifiable to pay for a journal or spend time in further reading, factors such as where the paper was published, by whom and when, should be evaluated. Ideally, data from *peer-reviewed journals* which have an *impact factor* should be sourced. The authors should be considered in terms of if they are the appropriate people to write about the topic and if they themselves would be a source of *bias*. Finally, considering when the paper was published and if the topic has evolved since is also important as this may also change the value of the information provided to your question. Once this information is established and the researcher is confident in the paper's credentials, the abstract should be reviewed.

The abstract is a summary of the research being presented. It should never be used alone without reading the rest of the paper as this can lead to significant omissions. However, it can tell you if you should read on or if you should move on. The abstract should always be read with the research question in mind and with consideration as to how this paper will help to answer it.

One of the first considerations when reading the abstract should be whether the article contains *primary*, *secondary*, or *tertiary* data. Clinical answers should only rely on primary data; however, secondary and tertiary can still be utilised to gain an understanding of the topic. Much of the published work in veterinary nursing falls into the secondary or tertiary categories combined with opinion, tradition, and/or experience, demonstrating the need for veterinary nurses to begin to undertake research to enable evidence-based practice.

Qualitative research may differ in the presentation of the abstract compared to quantitative and each journal will set author guidelines as to what should be covered in the abstract. However, the significant details regarding the background of the study, the research question, the methodology, the results, and the discussion should be evident. For each part of the abstract, the reader should be considering the *validity*, *reliability*, and *generalisability* of research they are presented with.

Not all papers should be discarded if they do not directly relate to the question, as information may still be gleaned from them. For example, a paper may be found that explores catheter tape in cats and whilst this does not answer the research question, it may help to demonstrate a valid and reliable method of collecting the data that can be applied to dogs. However, again, the clinical researcher should consider the worth of the paper to their question.

Critiquing the Research Paper

A good understanding of the research process aids the critical analysis process of the abstract, and the remainder of the research paper. This chapter focuses on how research should be structured and the factors to consider throughout, therefore reading the remaining sections may be used to build knowledge, understanding, and experience which can then be applied to a critique of a paper.

RCVS Knowledge have also provided a range of resources, EBVM Toolkits, 3–15 (RCVS Knowledge 2021e), regarding this aspect of research, including checklists, which can be particularly useful to ensure that each paper is approached with the same level of rigour. There are also many open access resources for veterinary and medical nurses, which follow similar principles. Again, the focus is the reliability, generalisability, and validity of the work in relation to the research question.

You may now wish to complete Exercise 9.5 and create your own critiquing process.

Answering the Question

Once the literature has been critiqued the clinical researcher must decide if they can fully answer their question.

If the question has been fully answered then the data search is completed, and the results found in the literature review can be applied to clinical practice. However, the clinical researcher may decide to write up their findings either as a literature review or as a critically appraised topic, both of which are widely published within veterinary nursing. Full author guidelines can be gained from the website of the journal that you wish to publish in and if a logical approach to the process thus far was taken, it would not take a considerable amount of time to restructure the findings to the required format.

Additionally, if the results were applied within the practice environment, the clinical researcher should audit the outcomes of this change as depicted in Figure 9.2.

Alternatively, if the question was not answered, only partially answered, answered with data demonstrating weak reliability, validity or generalisability, or the question has evolved since the data was published, the clinical researcher should start to consider collecting their own data to answer their clinical questions as described by the next section of this chapter.

Devising a Clinical Study

When devising a clinical study, the ideas driven from a practice-based question are transformed into something that can be measured and implemented. Planning how the study will be carried out is fundamental to producing results that are reliable and meaningful to clinical practice.

It is good practice to produce a *project proposal*. This helps the researcher implement their study design in clinical practice, and if carried out alongside nursing duties, it can be presented to an employer to show its value and the beneficial use of the employee's time. This sub-chapter will guide a novice researcher through the planning and implementation of a clinical study, considering each stage of the process though the project proposal.

Audit Versus Research

Before detailing the study design, it is beneficial to understand the difference between research and audit. Whilst they are interlinked and intrinsically influence changes in clinical practice based on the concepts of EBVN, they follow different processes and have different outcomes.

A clinical audit aims to review if best practice is being followed or if the best quality of care is being provided within a veterinary practice, typically through measuring processes, systems, and patient outcomes to highlight areas for improvement based on the outcome of the audit and published evidence. RCVS Knowledge (2019a) has outlined the clinical audit cycle and provided an audit template (RCVS Knowledge 2019b). In contrast, clinical research aims to generate new knowledge and provide new insights into the best quality of care through a systematic enquiry (Viner 2009).

Clinical audits are always observational by design, meaning that the researcher takes a passive role in 'observing' the outcome(s) of an intervention or exposure (e.g. surgical procedure) within a group of subjects (Katz 2006; Mosedale 2019). Current protocols, treatments, or patient care are measured to determine their clinical effectiveness as part of a quality improvement process. This would be within a veterinary practice or group of practices at an individual, team, or service level.

Clinical research may be either observational or experimental. Experimental studies involve the researcher playing an active role in designing an intervention (e.g. a diet change) and assigning which subjects will receive the intervention.

Both audits and clinical research can be further subdivided into a range of methodologies, as demonstrated in Figure 9.5. There is no one study design that is better than the others, and some more extensive clinical questions can be answered by using more than one design in succession. The best study design is the one that feasibly, reliably, efficiently, and ethically answers the study objective.

Some of the practical considerations for RVNs carrying out a clinical study are shown in Figure 9.6.

Project Proposal Step 1: Determine What Is Being Measured (Methodology)

A common pitfall when designing a clinical study is trying to answer too many questions at once. A simple study will address an elemental question or objective, using an appropriate methodology to justify the method of data collection. Time should be spent planning the study with enough information and detail to ensure that the study could be read and replicated by another researcher or auditor.

Defining an Aim and Objective

Once the general purpose of the study has been established through an exploration of the evidence, this should be written in the proposal as a broad statement of intent, known as the 'aim'. For example, the aim might be to *establish which catheter tape to use in canine patients*. The objective states *how* this will be achieved; for example, in a clinical audit, you may wish to review the number of patients that were recorded to have skin irritation on their practice records after a particular tape was used. A research-based objective would focus on finding out novel information about the use of a particular catheter tape by examining the

Type of clinical study	Description	Example	Application
Research: Experimental	Experimental research investigates a cause and effect relationship. The researcher designs the intervention (e.g. treatment) and assigns animals to be exposed/not exposed to it.	Question: Is physiotherapy treatment associated with a faster recovery time? The subjects are assigned to two groups: Physiotherapy received/not received	Generates new knowledge about best practice that can be used in EVBN to improve patient care.
Research: Observational	Observational research investigates relationships between variables by observing an intervention or exposure (e.g. surgical procedure) and its outcome within a group of animals.	Question: Is skin irritation associated with the type of intravenous catheter tape?	Generates new knowledge about best practice that can be used in EVBN to improve patient care.
Outcome audit	An outcome audit looks at the patient outcomes from the care/treatment/procedure given.	Question: How many postoperative complications following neutering are recorded? Can they be reduced?	An overview of patient care, that can be compared to a evidence-based target and the care improved.
Process audit	A process audit looks at whether the VPs protocols and guidelines are being followed correctly.	Question: Is a hand hygiene protocol being followed by practice staff?	An overview of how clinical care is being delivered. Highlights protocols and guidelines that can be implemented or improved.
Structure audit	A structure audit looks at the facilities and equipment in the veterinary practice (VP), i.e. What is being used and are they where they are needed.	Question: Are 'in-house' aural cytology swabs being taken for all ear exams before and after the prescribing of antibiotics?	Highlight's facilities and equipment that are not being used or the need for additional resources.
Significant event audit	A significant event audit looks at one specific event in detail to see what can be learnt (i.e., Part of a root-cause analysis when the impact of care has been negative).	Question: What can we learn from this specific case? Is there a safer way to deliver the care? i.e., when an incorrect medication has been dispensed to a patient.	Highlights protocols, guidelines and checklists that can be implemented or improved to increase positive patient outcomes or decrease negative patient outcomes.

Figure 9.5 Types of clinical study design. Source: Adapted from Mosedale (2020), RCVS Knowledge (2021g), NICE (2002).

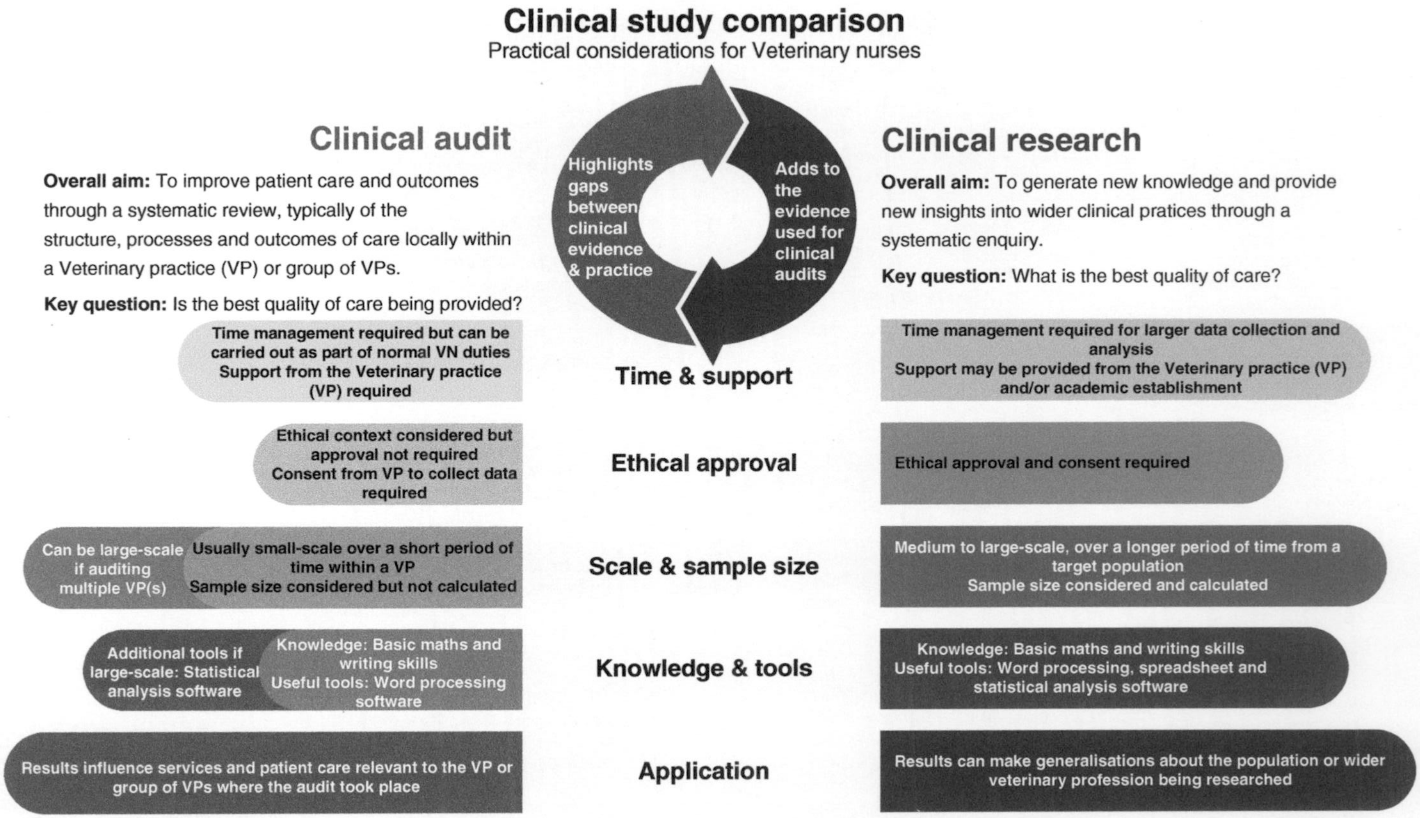

Clinical study comparison

Practical considerations for Veterinary nurses

Clinical audit

Overall aim: To improve patient care and outcomes through a systematic review, typically of the structure, processes and outcomes of care locally within a Veterinary practice (VP) or group of VPs.

Key question: Is the best quality of care being provided?

Clinical research

Overall aim: To generate new knowledge and provide new insights into wider clinical pratices through a systematic enquiry.

Key question: What is the best quality of care?

Highlights gaps between clinical evidence & practice

Adds to the evidence used for clinical audits

Time & support

Time management required but can be carried out as part of normal VN duties
Support from the Veterinary practice (VP) required

Time management required for larger data collection and analysis
Support may be provided from the Veterinary practice (VP) and/or academic establishment

Ethical approval

Ethical context considered but approval not required
Consent from VP to collect data required

Ethical approval and consent required

Scale & sample size

Can be large-scale if auditing multiple VP(s)

Usually small-scale over a short period of time within a VP
Sample size considered but not calculated

Medium to large-scale, over a longer period of time from a target population
Sample size considered and calculated

Knowledge & tools

Additional tools if large-scale: Statistical analysis software

Knowledge: Basic maths and writing skills
Useful tools: Word processing software

Knowledge: Basic maths and writing skills
Useful tools: Word processing, spreadsheet and statistical analysis software

Application

Results influence services and patient care relevant to the VP or group of VPs where the audit took place

Results can make generalisations about the population or wider veterinary profession being researched

Figure 9.6   Clinical study comparison between an audit and research. Modified and adapted from Wylie (2015).

relationship between the skin irritation reported and the type of tape used. It is usual to write the aims and objective together, for example;

- Clinical audit aim and objective: **To establish which catheter tape to use in canine patients** *by reviewing how many canine patients are reported to have skin irritation after a particular catheter tape was used.*
- Clinical research aim and objective: **To establish which catheter tape to use in canine patients** *by determining if there is an association between patient interference and skin irritation comparing two types of catheter tape in canine patients. (i.e. Determine if tape one or tape two causes more skin irritation and patient interference).*

(aim in bold, objective in italic).

It is normal to write several iterations of the study's objective to define it with measurable criteria/variables. These variables must be quantifiable, meaning they can be physically measured by collecting information.

Defining a Hypothesis

A hypothesis is a prediction of what you think the outcome of the study will be, it is used to express the effect, relationship, or difference between two *variables. Inferential statistics* are used in the analysis phase to test if there is *statistical significance* between the variables being measured or if any differences or association that were found occurred due to chance. The results mean that inferences or generalisations can be made about the study population (Maltby et al. 2007). A clinical audit does not require hypotheses, as it is observational and uses performance data to improve clinical practice, therefore relationships between variables are not being tested.

Setting a Clinical Target

Setting a target identifies the clinical relevance of the study and demonstrates how the work carried out contributes to improving care or making recommendations for improved care.

In clinical audits, the target is a desired improvement to patient care based on the best available evidence. Improvements should be aligned with guidelines or standards created by experts in their field and based on published evidence. They can be used to set and maintain target levels of care within a branch, a chain, or externally in the veterinary profession (NICE 2021; Benjamin 2008). In the absence of published guidelines or standards, it is recommended that practices run an initial audit to set a baseline level and use this as a future standard to audit against. This can be used in conjunction with the best evidence available to set clinical targets relevant to the veterinary practice (Waine and Brennan 2015).

Practices can also use benchmarks to determine if they can improve the quality of veterinary care. Benchmarks reflect current activity in veterinary care, highlighting how clinical activity in a veterinary practice compares to the national metrics. Benchmarking is extensively reported in the medical profession, but databases are currently being expanded in the veterinary profession (RCVS Knowledge 2020c). Examples of national databases include RVC VetCompass, holding data on common disorders such as corneal ulcer disease, hypoadrenocortism, and dystocia in dogs (RVC 2021), and RCVS National Audit for small animal neutering, which holds clinical activity on postoperative complications in routine neutering of dogs and cats (vetAUDIT 2021).

In clinical research, a target might include the methods of disseminating the outcome of the study to the wider veterinary community (e.g. publication in a journal or speaking at a conference) or post-research tools, guidelines or standards that may be developed because of the research. This also demonstrates the value of the research to stakeholders, as well as building the 'body of evidence' for EBVN.

It would be beneficial to now complete Exercise 9.6.

Choosing your Methodology

In defining your aims, objective, hypotheses, and target, you should have a good understanding of your study's outcomes and can therefore decide if you are undertaking an audit or research. Additionally, you should now have a better understanding of what type of data you are collecting, for example quantitative or qualitative, and therefore your *methodology*.

Project Proposal Step 2: Planning the Data Collection (Methods)

A fundamental part of the planning process is to decide; who the data will be collected from, what data will be collected and how it will be collected?

Identify the Target Population and Sample Population

In any research, it is impossible to sample the entire population (e.g. all cats), because it is too large and unknown, or samples may be collected from cats that are not the target of the study, which would be unethical. Therefore, a target population (e.g. owned cats in the U.K.) is used to target subjects that it is possible to sample. This is also the population that the outcome of the research will apply to, which will vary depending on the context of the research.

However, the target population may still be large (e.g. owned cats in the UK). Therefore, a sample population can be selected from the target population (e.g. owned cats in the UK that are vaccinated). This needs to be considered carefully, as the sample should accurately represent the population if the outcome is to make generalisations about that population. For example, if the target population is *owned cats in the UK that are vaccinated*, the sample should represent the sub-groups of this population (i.e. all types of age, sex, breed, etc.). It is worthwhile employing a sampling strategy to ensure a representative sample is recruited to the study (Katz 2006). *This is further explored in the online resources.*

Sample Size

Sample size is frequently discussed when critically appraising research for validity. The sample size relates to the precision of the study and whether it can be used to draw accurate conclusions about the target population.

To determine the minimum number of animals/participants that are needed to detect a statistically significant relationship/effect, a power calculation can be carried out using a free online tool, for example Select Statistical Services (2021). Whilst a larger sample size will yield greater precision and accuracy in the research analysis, it is worth considering the time, costs, feasibility, and ethical implications (particularly with experimental studies) of collecting more data than needed and therefore producing *research waste.*

Variables

Variables are the measurable factors in a study, they are what your method collects data on and are described in a study's objectives to examine how they relate to each other (Maltby et al. 2007; Leard statistics 2013).

Variables can change the outcome of the study and they can be manipulated or controlled as required for the question. Variables can be divided into variable types, and it is important to understand the difference between them for data analysis. The first difference relates to how the variables affect each other; known as *dependent* and *independent variables.* An independent variable (experimental variable) can be manipulated or observed so the researcher can measure the effect on a dependent variable (outcome variable) (Leard statistics 2013). Figure 9.7 details the variables for the catheter tape example. The independent variable is the type of catheter tape, the researcher can classify the groups of patients according to the tape applied for catheter placement. The researcher could either assign patients to

Variable type	Example	
Independent (experimental)	Type of catheter tape:	Tape 1
		Tape 2
Dependent (outcome)	1) Skin irritation	
	2) Patient interference	

Figure 9.7   Examples of independent and dependents variables. Source: Based on Leard statistics 2013.

Variable category	Variable sub-category	Example
Categorical (Qualitative categories)	Nominal – Two or more separate categories	Breed of dog: Labrador, Dalmatian, Boxer
	Ordinal – Two or more ordered categories	Level of pain in dogs: Mild, moderate, severe
	Dichotomous – Two mutually exclusive categories	Vaccination status: Vaccinated or unvaccinated
Numerical (Quantitative categories)	Continuous – Can be measured along a numerical continuum (i.e. continuous scale). The data collected can have decimal places.	Body temperature of a dog: 38.3 degrees Celsius
	Discrete – Can be measured in whole numerical terms.	Number of puppies: 0, 1, 2, 3... 15

Figure 9.8   Examples of variable categories and sub-categories. Source: Information from Leard Statistics (2013).

a catheter tape group (experiential study) or randomly select patients from the population of dogs that received tape one or tape two (observational study). The dependent variable is therefore skin irritation and patient interference, as these are the possible outcomes of using different tapes.

Further division of the independent and dependent variables separates their characteristics. Categorical variables are those that can be categorised in a qualitative way and can be sub divided into nominal, ordinal, and dichotomous categories. Numerical variables are those that can be quantified in numbers; they are sub-divided into continuous and discrete categories as described in Figure 9.8. It is important to know these for data analysis and to understand how you are going to collect that data.

Method Types

Methods are the tools used to collect the data. Where possible it is beneficial to utilise pre-existing validated tools (e.g. pain scale) or tools that have been used in other studies and have been proven to reliably collect the data required. Again, the clinical researcher must review the question and what it is trying to answer to decide the best method for their study.

Data may be collected either retrospectively (data that already exists) or prospectively (data that is collected at the time) and the literature review may demonstrate a range of appropriate methods. These may include quantitative methods or qualitative methods. Any prospective methods should be *piloted* prior to use to ensure they collect the required data in a reliable and user-friendly manner.

Quantitative methods include the collection of data from patient care forms, checklists, patient records, anaesthetic monitoring forms, retrospectively, or prospectively for example, via questionnaires designed specifically for the research in either paper or electronic form.

Qualitative methods include those which allow for qualities or characteristics to be described. This is usually collected in a narrative form through questionnaires, interviews, or focus groups. Examples of this data type include describing animal behaviour or understanding the opinions of a focus group discussing animal welfare. There are many other resources that describe qualitative study design further, such as those described by Clarke and Braun (2013) and Ingham-Broomfield (2014).

You may now wish to complete Exercise 9.7.

Project Proposal Step 3: Implementing Data Collection

There are some practical considerations (see Figure 9.9) which must relate to the scope and scale of the intended research. The lead researcher should plan the data collection with a critical eye and look for potential problems that could hinder the research or data collection itself. If the data is being collected prospectively in clinical practice, it is usual for the researcher to lead, but it does not mean that they need to collect it all themselves. With adequate training in the method, the veterinary team can support the lead researcher.

Research Ethics

Veterinary nurses enter the profession to maintain and improve the welfare of animals, it is essential that this also extends to research that they may conduct or participate in. However, research ethics are not limited to the patient, but incorporate the client, the veterinary team, and the handling of data.

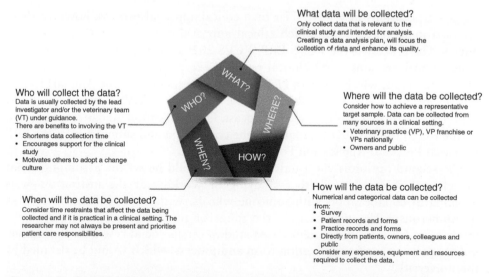

What data will be collected?
Only collect data that is relevant to the clinical study and intended for analysis. Creating a data analysis plan, will focus the collection of data and enhance its quality.

Who will collect the data?
Data is usually collected by the lead investigator and/or the veterinary team (VT) under guidance.
There are benefits to involving the VT
• Shortens data collection time
• Encourages support for the clinical study
• Motivates others to adopt a change culture

Where will the data be collected?
Consider how to achieve a representative target sample. Data can be collected from many sources in a clinical setting.
• Veterinary practice (VP), VP franchise or VPs nationally
• Owners and public

When will the data be collected?
Consider time restraints that affect the data being collected and if it is practical in a clinical setting. The researcher may not always be present and prioritise patient care responsibilities.

How will the data be collected?
Numerical and categorical data can be collected from:
• Survey
• Patient records and forms
• Practice records and forms
• Directly from patients, owners, colleagues and public
Consider any expenses, equipment and resources required to collect the data.

Figure 9.9   Considerations for veterinary nurses on practice-based data collection.

The Requirement for Ethical Approval

All research conducted must be ethical. Research that breaks ethical conventions will meet with disapproval from the profession, the governing body, and any potential publishers. Furthermore, it may lead to the researcher breaching legislation and codes of professional conduct, which both have their own serious implications. However, many of the principles of ethical research are within the Code of Professional Conduct for veterinary nurses (RCVS Knowledge 2016) and are aligned to the care of animals and the service provided to owners. Therefore, the clinical researcher can consider these factors in the process of data collection.

Gaining approval from an ethical review panel (ERP) means that a committee of experienced peers have considered the study and agreed that ethical boundaries will be maintained during the project. This provides a novice researcher with confidence that someone with greater experience in research methods and research legislation has reviewed and approved the proposal presented (RCVS 2021).

Research studies require ethical approval to review a change or a comparison in patient care, which may have an unknown or negative effect on the participant. Audits are less likely to require ethical approval as the normal level of care for the patient or service to the client remains unchanged. If ethical approval has not been sought, the researcher must still gain consent from the practice to use the data. However, most publishers would expect ethical approval to be present within any submission and may not publish the research in their journal without it and it is now certainly an expectation of the profession (RCVS Knowledge 2016).

Seeking Ethical Approval

Large corporations may have their own ethical approval process, however, there are two main places from which ethical approval can be sought by veterinary nurses. The first is via the RCVS ERP (RCVS 2020a). This panel will consider the ethical considerations of all clinical research except those deemed to be experimental research, which requires Home Office licensing under the Animals (Scientific Procedures) Act 1986 (RCVS 2019). Mellanby (RCVS Knowledge 2016) explores this further in a free access podcast. Full application guidance is provided by the RCVS (RCVS 2020b), requiring the completion and submission of the ERP Research Proposal Application Form (RCVS 2021).

The second option is via a university. This would be on the assumption that the clinical researcher is either studying or working at the institution or is working in collaboration with someone who is. Within universities, there may be numerous ERPs, which cover the range of research conducted within the institution, for example patient-based studies versus social research. Each panel may require a specific application form and process, which would be detailed by the university.

If ethical approval is granted, the researcher will be supplied with a code referencing the successful application, which is then reported when the work is published within the methods section.

Considerations of Practice-Based Research

The key factors that ERPs consider is whether the research is required, if the methodology and methods used are justifiable and will not cause harm and if those recruited to the study have provided informed consent. This therefore requires details of the background of the project, the research question, aims, objectives, and hypotheses, the methods, the potential analysis plan, any incentives for participation and, importantly, the ethical considerations of the study and the approach taken to minimise their impact.

General, but crucial factors to consider for both research and audits are:

- *Data handling:* Data protection must be maintained throughout; veterinary nurses must ensure they follow GDPR 2018 and the Data Protection Act 2018. The Caldicott Principles for patient information can be used to guide this aspect of the research (depicted in Figure 9.10).
- *Informed consent:* Owners must be fully informed about the research and must have been provided with the opportunity to consider the information, ask questions and provide consent. The information sheet and consent form should detail the purpose of the study, the methods, who the researchers are, and if the project has received funding. If the owner does not consent, then there should be no ramifications of this nor should there be if the participant withdraws at any time during the study. Again, clear information must be provided on how to do this.
- *Legislation:* Veterinary nurses should have a good understanding of the Animals (Scientific Procedures) Act 1986, in addition to the requirement for an Animal Test Certificate (GOV.UK 2015) and Animal Welfare Act 2006, so that an informed decision can be made as to whether additional requirements are

---

1. One should justify the purpose of holding patient information.
2. Information on patients should only be held if absolutely necessary.
3. Use only the minimum of information that is required.
4. Information access should be on a strict need to know basis.
5. Everyone in the organisation should be aware of their responsibilities.
6. The organisation should understand and comply with the law.

(The Caldicott Committee, 1997)

Figure 9.10   The Caldicott Principles. Source: Adapted from The Caldicott Committee, 1997.

needed for the research. This would be flagged at the ethical approval panel; however, awareness of this prior to submission may save time. Some guidance is provided by the RCVS on the requirements for a Home Office licence under the Animals (Scientific Procedures) Act 1986 (RCVS 2019).

• *Integrity:* the clinical researcher should act with integrity throughout, they should maintain the methodology and methods, remain open and honest, and conduct the research with rigour. If complications arise or changes are made to the study, the ERP must be informed.

There is also a range of ethical frameworks available which may help to guide the clinical researcher. Two useful frameworks are the Beauchamp and Childress's (2001) four principles of biomedical ethics and Russel and Burch's (1959) 3 Rs. The Beauchamp and Childress model (2001) is useful for both research and audits, whereas Russel and Burch's 3 Rs is more likely to be used in the planning of research as the focus is on reducing the impact of research on participants.

You may now wish to undertake Activity 8; this will be a useful exercise for all to apply knowledge and understanding.

Undertaking the Study

Once the methodology has been decided and ethical approval gained, data collection can begin. At this stage being organised is key. If an issue occurs, for example it becomes apparent that the method is not allowing the appropriate collection of data the project should be halted. If changes are required, the ethical approval panel must be updated, and the study should only resume once this has been re-approved. Any data collected prior to this issue may have to be discarded as it will no longer be comparable to the data following the intervention.

Making Sense of the Data – Analysis and Interpretation

Approach to Data Analysis

Those who are new to clinical studies may have some trepidations about analysing their data, but this is the point when all the time and planning put in at the beginning of the process comes to fruition. Before starting the analysis, it is helpful to revisit the aims and objectives, which will focus the approach taken.

The approach to analysis will depend on the size and scale of the study, but also whether the study is a clinical audit or research. The analysis can involve calculating *descriptive statistics* or include more complex *inferential statistics*. The information presented on this topic here is simplified and tailored for novice researchers. There are many online resources on data analysis which explore the principles and execution in further detail.

Organising and Storing Data

The initial outcome of all clinical studies is data. It is beneficial to organise the data from its raw state (i.e. patient records, monitoring form, checklist, or questionnaire) by putting it into a *spreadsheet*. This has several advantages, as the data can be:

- analysed in a manageable and logical way.
- stored appropriately for future use (i.e. compared with data from a re-audit if there is consent to do so)
- analysed using inferential statistics (clinical research data).

Data management software is widely accepted as a simple, logical, and time-saving tool for organising and analysing data. Most practices will have access to common data spreadsheets (i.e. Microsoft Excel® or Mac Numbers®) which allow descriptive statistics to be performed. If the data has been collected from Practice Management Systems it can often be exported directly to a spreadsheet for analysis. At this point data may be anonymised, for example via the application of a unique number for each individual participant, and the document should be password-protected.

Once the data is in a spreadsheet, it can be 'cleaned'. This can be achieved in several ways:

- Dealing with missing data or incomplete responses – this can occur when you, other members of the veterinary team, or owners are inputting the data, for example missing questions within a questionnaire. This is frustrating, but the researcher must decide how significant the missing data is to the study's objective and whether the data collected for that patient/respondent should be omitted completely or just for a single question.
- Checking data entry is uniform – if the same word can be written in multiple ways, the entry must be the same throughout the spreadsheet. For example, domestic short hair should be written in full or as DSH.

Data Analysis: Descriptive Statistics

Descriptive statistics are techniques that help to interpret and display the data collected in a study. As veterinary professionals, nurses are regularly presented with descriptive statistics, for example mortality rates or average recovery times, and use them frequently to make clinical judgements about how we or our team provide care to patients (Maltby et al. 2007).

Creating an analysis plan in the form of a table, can be beneficial to organise variables. In the first column, each variable should be placed into a row, then in the second column the type of variable should be listed. Following this, the third column should state the descriptive technique that will be utilised as described in the following section.

Categorical Variables

Frequencies

At the beginning of any clinical study report the frequency of the variables should be summarised. This is the number of subjects or number of times an event occurred (Maltby et al. 2007) both as a total number and as a percentage. It is important to record both number and percentage, as whilst the percentage is an easier number to understand, it can be misleading. For example, if a study reported a 50% complication rate for a catheter tape, the value that is attributed to that finding would vary greatly if the study only sampled two dogs, versus two hundred.

A frequency table can be utilised to display this information, for example Figure 9.11. In this scenario, 200 dogs were sampled and the RVN recorded how many of those patients had either 'Skin irritation' or 'No skin irritation'. This was recorded in terms of the number of samples (patient participants) in each category and the percentage expressed as the proportion of that variable within that category (i.e. 120 dogs are 60% of the sample of 200).

You can find numerous percentage calculators online if you search for *percentage calculator*. However, you can also do this simple calculation for frequency proportion without digital assistance by calculating:

Frequency number within the category ÷ Total number reported for that variable = Frequency

Frequency $\times 100$ = Frequency proportion

$$E.g. 120(\text{dogs : no skin irritation}) \div 200(\text{total number dogs}) = 0.6(\text{frequency})$$

$$0.6 \times 100 = 60\% \ (\text{frequency proportion})$$

Presentation of Information

As stated throughout this chapter, data collected should be disseminated. Some will find it easier to report the numbers in their spreadsheet prior to writing descriptively about the data, whilst others will feel more comfortable writing the variable as a sentence. Reviewing other published studies can be beneficial to

Skin condition	Frequency of dogs	Percentage of dogs (%)
No skin irritation	120	60
Skin irritation	80	40

Figure 9.11   Reported skin condition in dogs (N = 200) who received the new intravenous catheter tape.

understand the different ways this may be achieved. Tables can be used to demonstrate the information but should be given context with a sentence or two. A common way of summarising the table above could be:

'Two hundred dogs were sampled, and out of those participants, 60% (N = 120) had no skin irritation from the catheter tape and 40% (N = 80) were found to have skin irritation'.

Note that both percentage and number, presented as N =, are provided, but so is the total number of participants in that variable. The latter is important because, as previously mentioned, there may be gaps in the data set from an individual response.

Numeric Variables

Numeric variables are handled differently to categorical variables, as the analysis of data deals with numbers rather than categories and how these numbers are distributed within a data set.

Measures of Tendency

To demonstrate where the data set tends to cluster around, i.e. the most common point, you need to look at either the *mean* or *median* of the values. This is called the central tendency, in other words, what was the most common value. When deciding whether mean or median is utilised you must again go back to the data. Mean, the average of all the numbers, is useful when a roughly equal proportion of the data is distributed either side of that central point. However, if more of the data are distributed towards one end of the scale, the average can become *skewed* and it is therefore not representative of the central point of the data.

A hypothetical data set is presented in Figure 9.12. In group a, the ages are mostly in the centre of the minimum and maximum value in the data collected, and there is an equal spread around that central point, whereas in b, most of the cats are younger. If b were to be plotted on a graph, it would be skewed as per Figure 9.13, and this causes the average age to skew. Median, the middle value of all the numbers, is beneficial in this instance because the median of data set b would be one, which is, again, more representative of the central point of the data.

Cat group	Data set age (years)					Mean	Median
a	1	3	3	3	5	3	3
b	1	1	1	3	5	2	1

Figure 9.12   Hypothetical data set for central point.

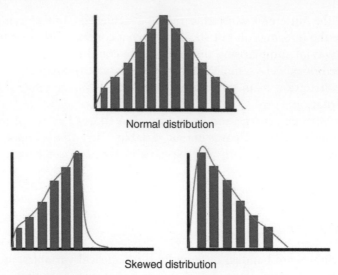

Normal distribution

Skewed distribution

Figure 9.13   Data distribution shapes.

When data are clustered around the central point and have a roughly equal distribution either side, it is called *normal distribution*, and mean is used to describe the data. When data are clustered around a point that is either higher or lower than the middle value, then they are *not normally distributed*, and median is used to describe the data.

To decide upon the normality of data a *histogram* should be created. The data should be plotted, and then a line drawn joining the top of the points. If a bell shape is seen as depicted by Figure 9.13, it is normally distributed. If it slopes away from the centre, again depicted in Figure 9.13, then it is not normally distributed.

Many spreadsheets allow the creation of histograms. This can be used to gauge the overall shape. There are also statistical analysis software packages that can calculate this, if the clinical researcher has access to such software. Again, there are many free video tutorials online for both approaches. Furthermore, this is where approaching an experienced mentor is beneficial, as they may be able to support you in this process or have the required software.

Measures of Variability

After finding the value that the data cluster around, it is important to know the *range* of that data. This is the measure of variability, how much do the results vary from that central figure. If the data are normally distributed, *Standard Deviation* should be used. If the data are not normally distributed, then the minimum and maximum value should be provided.

The minimum and maximum can be easily viewed within smaller data sets. However, there are also functions within spreadsheets such as Microsoft® Excel®

(Microsoft Corporation, 2022) which can be used to identify these. Likewise, standard deviation can be calculated within spreadsheets and full instructions can be found online and followed for both functions. Data analysis software programs such as IBM® SPSS® (IBM corp. SPSS, 2022) or R® (R Core Team, 2022) can also identify these measures, and there are numerous video tutorials and resources online which can take you through the process of calculating these descriptive statistics.

Presentation of Information

The data should be summarised in a short sentence such as 'the median age of cats that were vaccinated was 10, (2–15)'. Again, reviewing published journals can demonstrate how this may be presented within a full research report. '2–15' describes the minimum and maximum value.

Graphs

Graphs help to visually demonstrate the meaning of the results without comprehensive explanation, provided the axes and title are appropriately labelled. They can be generated from a spreadsheet or statistical program. There are many types of graph and the type of graph will depend on the variables and purpose. For example, pie charts can help to demonstrate proportions at a glance, which is useful for a poster, but specific details are less clear and therefore they are generally not used in journal publications, where the readers are likely to want greater detail. Generally, *bar charts, histograms, scatterplots,* or *box and whisker plots* are used. *Please see the companion website for more information on presenting data in graphs.*

Reporting the Results

The data for each variable collected should be described, and no variables should be omitted as the data was collected for a purpose in answering the clinical question. At this point, for audits and research projects that do not have hypotheses, the statistical analysis is complete. However, for hypothesis-driven studies, inferential statistics are still required.

Data Analysis: Inferential Statistics

Inferential statistics can be used to draw *inferences* or make conclusions about the population. It uses probability to determine the strength of evidence that conclusions are correct. Therefore, this can help determine how strong a possibility it is that differences, effects, or associations between variables occurred due to chance. For example, if three catheter tapes were used in a study and tape 1 seemed to have far more patients in the category of 'skin irritation', inferential statistics can help to show if that was a true association (catheter tape 1 is more likely to cause irritation than tape 2 or 3), or if the difference found was just caused by chance.

The variables that should be tested are those described in the hypothesis. It is not acceptable to test other random variables to search for opportunistic links. Having a clear idea as to which variables you would like to test in this manner is key to answering your aims, objectives, and research question.

There are numerous statistical analysis tests for different: types of variables, number of variables, type of association and data distribution. For example, data that is normally distributed uses *parametric tests* and data that is not normally distributed uses *non-parametric tests*. These are explored further in the *companion website* as it is beyond the scope of this chapter to explore each method of analysis and how they are conducted.

It is usual to conduct these tests in statistical analysis software such as IBM® SPSS® Statistics which is a powerful statistical software program that allows the researcher to organise, represent and analyse data (IMB corp. SPSS, 2022) or R®, an open-source programming language and free software program that allows statistical inference and analysis (R Core Team, 2022). Both offer analytical tools and can be used to organise data from a spreadsheet, generate graphs and analyse data.

Ultimately, the result of statistical analysis is a '*p value*'. The p stands for probability, the probability of any associations or differences occurring due to chance. Most studies will report 'p ≤0.05'. This means that if the p value is less than or equal to 0.05, the difference or association found is statistically significant and there is only a 5% (or lower) risk that this occurred due to chance.

No test will ever confirm 100% association and therefore, when writing up results following hypothesis testing, one must be careful not to state this assumption. To write up this section, you must refer to your descriptive statistics of the variables tested for the hypothesis and then state whether any associations or differences found were truly occurring or due to chance. For example, if your research question was; Is there any difference in skin irritation between catheter tape 1 and catheter tape 2? The hypothesis might be: 'There is an association between skin irritation in patients and catheter tape' or 'Skin irritation in patients differs between catheter tapes 1 and 2'. If there is statistical significance, the p value will be less than or equal to 0.05 (p≤0.05). The researcher could then write the results as:

> Eighty percent (N = 375) of patients with catheter tape 1 had skin irritation versus 35% (N = 125) of those with catheter tape 2. This difference was found to be statistically significant p = 0.03 and therefore catheter tape 1 will be more likely to cause skin irritation in dogs, when securing intravenous catheters, than catheter tape 2.

If the p value is found to be greater than 0.05, any associations or differences found within the variables are considered to be not statistically significant. However, this is important to report as it is still of relevance to clinical practice. An association not being linked is just as important as one that is linked as it still tells you likely clinical outcomes.

When there are numerous categories within a variable, it is not always clear which of the variables is causing the statistically significant result. Therefore, *post hoc tests* are required. These are again completed within the data analysis software.

Reviewing published research studies is beneficial in order to see how this type of information is being presented. Some will discuss hypothesis and null hypothesis, whilst others will just use the former. Again, this is explored in specific resources for research methods, but for simplicity, the hypothesis is sufficient for novice researchers.

Interpreting the Data

Following the analysis of the data and the write-up of the results, the clinical researcher needs to begin to consider what all the data means. Before this point, data should only be reported, and no judgements made as per the example sentences provided earlier in this chapter.

However, in the discussion section of an audit and research report, the results should be explored in the context of the clinical question, the background of the study, the application to practice, and recommendations for changes that should occur based upon the outcome of the study.

The discussion should be supported with relevant studies comparing any similarities that increase the validity of the results and any differences as well as potential reasons for this. The clinical researcher should be critical of their study, being open and honest about any limitations and the extent to which this affects the validity, reliability, and generalisability of the results.

Finally, any remaining questions and future areas of study should be raised, and the report concluded with the key points and their application to practice.

Final Thoughts

In some instances, the study will not yield the results expected and you may even have more questions about the area investigated, in which case further research or an audit can be planned, as per Figure 9.2.

Dissemination and Using the Results to Improve Practice

The dissemination process starts during the formation of an enquiring question, when the veterinary nurse 'thinks' about how they can change the quality of patient care for the better (O'Neill 2017). EBVN is dependent upon clinical nurses investigating and addressing specific areas of patient care by using existing knowledge and adding new knowledge from their own clinical studies.

As discussed, research should not be conducted if it is not going to be shared with the stakeholders. However, there are additional benefits to publishing, shown in Figure 9.14.

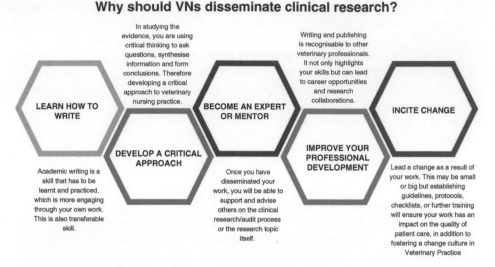

Why should VNs disseminate clinical research?

In studying the evidence, you are using critical thinking to ask questions, synthesise information and form conclusions. Therefore developing a critical approach to veterinary nursing practice.

Writing and publishing is recognisable to other veterinary professionals. It not only highlights your skills but can lead to career opportunities and research collaborations.

LEARN HOW TO WRITE

BECOME AN EXPERT OR MENTOR

INCITE CHANGE

DEVELOP A CRITICAL APPROACH

IMPROVE YOUR PROFESSIONAL DEVELOPMENT

Academic writing is a skill that has to be learnt and practiced, which is more engaging through your own work. This is also transferable skill.

Once you have disseminated your work, you will be able to support and advise others on the clinical research/audit process or the research topic itself.

Lead a change as a result of your work. This may be small or big but establishing guidelines, protocols, checklists, or further training will ensure your work has an impact on the quality of patient care, in addition to fostering a change culture in Veterinary Practice

Figure 9.14　Why veterinary nurses should disseminate clinical research.

Disseminating the Research Findings

There are many ways to disseminate the findings of a clinical study. Depending on the target audience, the language and form of dissemination may change, so it is worth thinking about who your target audience are, for example, veterinary, or vet' nurse practitioners, veterinary, welfare or regulatory bodies, owners or the public, the wider scientific community.

Sharing Locally with the Veterinary Practice or Stakeholders

If your clinical study was driven from a practice-based clinical question, then it is likely that the results are valuable to the practice where the enquiry originated, as well as to other stakeholders involved in the study. There are numerous ways of sharing your findings with the clinical team, with permission from the practice, for example:

- practice meetings
- journal clubs
- in-house CPD
- newsletters
- email updates
- social media updates.

Discussions around this can then highlight changes for quality of care improvement or lead to further investigations within the team. It is good role modelling for others and, overall, aids quality improvement.

Sharing with a Wider Audience

O'Neill (2017) presents a clear example of how research can be effectively disseminated to a wider audience in an Open Access podcast (Veterinary Evidence), but some examples include:

- presenting a poster at a conference
- via educational seminars
- speaking on a podcast
- targeting owners and the public via infographic posters, display boards, leaflets, or educational videos
- organising an outreach event with owners or the local community
- sharing results with clinical trial databases (RCVS Knowledge 2021h)
- writing a journal article.

Publishing the findings in a clinically relevant journal will mean that those searching for answers to the same clinical question, can find the required results. Where possible, the study should be freely accessible to everyone to help other nurses with EBVN. However, there may be challenges associated with this, for example, this sometimes requires the author to pay to publish on that platform.

Audits and knowledge summaries can be published free on an open access platform such as RCVS Knowledge (RCVS Knowledge 2021f). However, it may be more relevant to the topic to publish with a journal that is not open access. Additionally, some veterinary nursing journals pay their authors and so, whilst the paper should be published on the forum where it will have the maximum impact and reach the greatest number of interested people, it is still a consideration, particularly if costs need to be recouped.

It is helpful to review other reports or publications relevant to the research topic and reflect on where they are published and the style in which they are written. Each journal will have its own author guidelines and/or, less frequently, a template to complete, found on their website. However, the structure of this chapter is the commonly expected format. This is known as the IMRaD format, Introduction (including the literature review), Methods, Results, and Discussion. Each publisher will also detail how the information should be submitted, often with a specific platform that they utilise for each journal. If there is a peer review process, it will also be detailed on the journal's website.

Following the submission of work to a journal, a decision is made on whether the work will be accepted. If the study is accepted, you should expect that there will be peer review comments to work through. A discussion on these can occur, but if a reviewer feels strongly about a point, it could prevent the study article from being accepted unless altered. Once accepted, the editorial team will guide you through the process.

It may take months from the submission of an article to be published in print, or online. As with all other steps, it is beneficial to have a mentor who will answer your questions and provide guidance and reassurance, particularly after receiving numerous revisions and recommended edits, which can commonly occur.

Improving Practice – the Impact of your Results

The dissemination of results has been advocated throughout this chapter. Publishing your work is a real achievement and it can bring a sense of pride to you, your colleagues, your practice, and the profession.

As RVNs, the key focus and impact of any clinical study is to encourage quality improvement; defined by Batalden and Davidoff (2007) as 'The combined and unceasing efforts of everyone to make the changes that will lead to better patient outcomes (health), better system performance (care) and better professional development (learning)'. The findings from your study may provide information that can be compared to the standards available or a pre-determined clinical target and therefore inform changes. It may reveal areas of less desirable practice, which can be dispelled, and be used to evidence better practice. This quality improvement is achieved by establishing or adapting aspects of patient care and processes of care, as well as developing understanding and fostering a positive change culture in practice. Examples of this are through:

- guidelines (for veterinary professionals, paraprofessionals, owners, or the public)
- checklists
- Standard Operating Procedures
- assessment forms
- providing additional training, and mentoring to staff
- investing in additional equipment, facilities, or staff.

There are many good resources available from RCVS Knowledge on quality improvement in veterinary practice that can be accessed free online (RCVS Knowledge 2020d).

Final Thoughts

Disseminating the findings of your study will drive you and others to implement changes to improve practice. The application of research is the last step in the evidence-based practice process and it is necessary for quality improvement. Clinical targets set in the planning phase of the study, should be revisited and actioned. The original question should also be reflected upon and any outstanding areas that have not been answered should be considered.

Although this is the end of the chapter, it is not the end of the journey. A clinical researcher should continue to assess and re-assess the outcomes of their study, re-auditing, researching, and collaborating with others to establish improvements and add to the evidence base.

Share your passion, keep asking questions and make your work count.

Now visit the companion website where you will find additional resources for this chapter: www.wiley.com/go/badger/professionalism-veterinary-nursing.

References

Batalden, P.B. and Davidoff, F. (2007). What is 'quality improvement' and how can it transform healthcare? *BMJ Qual. Saf.* 16: 2–3.

Beauchamp, T.L. and Childress, J.F. (2001). *Principles of Biomedical Ethics*, 5e. New York: Oxford University Press.

Benjamin, A. (2008). Audit: how to do it in practice. *BMJ* 336: 1241–1245. https://doi.org/10.1136/bmj.39527.628322.AD.

Clarke, V. and Braun, V. (2013). *Successful Qualitative Research: A Practical Guide for Beginners*. SAGE.

Doran, G.T. (1981). There's a S.M.A.R.T. way to write management's goals and objectives. *Manag. Rev.* 70 (11): 35–36.

Gibbs, G. (1988). *Learning by Doing: A Guide to Teaching and Learning Methods*. Oxford: Oxford Brooks University.

GOV.UK. (2015). Animal Test Certificate. https://www.gov.uk/guidance/animal-test-certificates (accessed18 March 2021).

S. Hauser and Jackson, E. (2017). A survey of the non-clinical benefits of EBVM. *Vet. Evid.* 2(3). https://doi.org/10.18849/ve.v2i3.102

IBM corp SPSS (2022) IBM SPSS Statistics for Windows: Version 27.0. Armonk, NY: IBM Corp. Avalible at: https://www.ibm.com/uk-en/products/spss-statistics (accessed: 7 April 2022).

Ingham-Broomfield, B. (2014). A nurses' guide to qualitative research. *Aust. J. Adv. Nurs.* 32: 34.

Katz, M. (2006). *Study Design and Statistical Analysis: A Practical Guide for Clinicians*. Cambridge: Cambridge University Press.

Kolb, D.A. (1984). *Experiential Learning: Experience as the Source of Learning and Development*. Englewood Cliffs, NJ: Prentice-Hall.

Leard statistics (2013). SPSS statistics: Types of variable. https://statistics.laerd.com/premium/spss/tov/types-of-variable.php (accessed: 20 March 2021).

Maltby, J., Day, L., and Williams, G. (2007). *Introduction to Statistics for Nurses*. Harlow, Routledge.

Microsoft Corporation (2022). Microsoft Excel, Available at: https://office.microsoft.com/excel. (Accessed: 7 April 2022).

Moody, C., Picketts, V.A., Mason, G. et al. (2018). Can you handle it? Validating negative responses to restraint in cats. *Appl. Anim. Behav. Sci.* 204: 94–100.

Mosedale, P. (2019). Clinical audit in veterinary practice – the role of the veterinary nurse. *The Veterinary Nurse* 10 (1): 4–10.

Mosedale, P. (2020). The different types of clinical audit and how to perform them. *In Pract.* 42: 581–584. https://doi.org/10.1136/inp.m4043.

NICE (2002). Principles for best practice in clinical audit. https://www.nice.org.uk/media/default/About/what-we-do/Into-practice/principles-for-best-practice-in-clinical-audit.pdf (accessed: 9 March 2021).

NICE (2021). Principles for putting evidence-based guidance into practice. https://intopractice.nice.org.uk/principles-putting-evidence-based-guidance-into-practice/index.html#group-commitment-to-quality-improvement-9YO6RQOANx. (accessed: 7 March 2021).

O'Neill, D. (2017). Effective dissemination – building an 'Evidence to Impact' strategy. *Vet. Evid.* 2 (1): https://doi.org/10.18849/ve.v2i1.

R Core Team (2022). R: A language and environment for statistical computing. R Foundation for Statistical Computing, Vienna, Austria. URL https://www.r-project.org/ (accesssed: 7 April 2022).

RCVS (2019). The Royal College of Veterinary Surgeons Ethics Review Panel: guidance notes for applicants. https://www.rcvs.org.uk/document-library/erp-research-proposal-application-guidelines (accessed 18 March 2021).

RCVS (2020a). Ethics Review Panel what is it and how did it come about? https://www.rcvs.org.uk/news-and-views/webinars-and-podcasts/ethics-review-panel-what-is-it-and-how-did-it-come-about (accessed 18 March 2021).

RCVS (2020b). ERP Research Proposal Application Guidelines. https://www.rcvs.org.uk/document-library/erp-research-proposal-application-guidelines (accessed 18 March 2021).

RCVS (2021). Ethics Review Panel. https://www.rcvs.org.uk/who-we-are/committees/standards-committee/ethics-review-panel (accessed 18 March 2021).

RCVS Knowledge (2016). Richard Mellanby – The only way is ethics? Undertaking research as a practice-based vet/RVN [podcast] https://rcvsknowledge.podbean.com/e/the-only-way-is-ethics-undertaking-research-as-a-practice-based-vetrvn (accessed 18 March 2021).

RCVS Knowledge (2019a). The clinical audit cycle. https://knowledge.rcvs.org.uk/document-library/the-clinical-audit-walkthrough (accessed: 10 March 2021).

RCVS Knowledge (2019b). The clinical audit template. https://knowledge.rcvs.org.uk/document-library/clinical-audit-template (accessed: 10 March 2021).

RCVS Knowledge (2020a). Tools to help you complete Significant Event Audit – Root cause analysis. https://knowledge.rcvs.org.uk/document-library/tools-to-help-you-complete-significant-event-audit (accessed: 9 March 2021).

RCVS Knowledge (2020b). EBVM Toolkit 2: Finding the best available evidence. https://knowledge.rcvs.org.uk/document-library/ebvm-toolkit-2-finding-the-best-available-evidence (accessed 14 March 2021).

RCVS Knowledge (2020c). Benchmarking https://knowledge.rcvs.org.uk/quality-improvement/tools-and-resources/benchmarking (accessed: 10 March 2021).

RCVS Knowledge (2020d). Quality improvement. https://knowledge.rcvs.org.uk/quality-improvement. (accessed 6 January 2022).

RCVS Knowledge (2021a). Knowledge summaries. https://knowledge.rcvs.org.uk/evidence-based-veterinary-medicine/knowledge-summaries (accessed: 9 March 2021).

RCVS Knowledge (2021b). How does EBVM affect me? https://knowledge.rcvs.org.uk/evidence-based-veterinary-medicine/what-is-ebvm/how-does-ebvm-affect-me (accessed: 9 March 2021).

RCVS Knowledge (2021c). What is EBVM? https://knowledge.rcvs.org.uk/evidence-based-veterinary-medicine/what-is-ebvm (accessed: 9 March 2021).

RCVS Knowledge (2021d). Our services. https://knowledge.rcvs.org.uk/library-and-information-services/our-services/#literature (accessed 14 March 2021).

RCVS Knowledge (2021e). EBVM toolkit. https://knowledge.rcvs.org.uk/evidence-based-veterinary-medicine/ebvm-toolkit/#critically (accessed 14 March 2021).

RCVS Knowledge (2021f). Guidelines for authors. https://veterinaryevidence.org/index.php/ve/guidelines-for-authors (accessed: 9 March 2021).

RCVS Knowledge (2021g). Types of clinical audit. https://oncourse.rcvsk.org/wp-content/uploads/sites/4/2018/11/017-Types-of-Audit-Flowchart.pdf (accessed 20 March 2021).

RCVS Knowledge (2021h). EVBM resources: Clinical research. https://knowledge.rcvs.org.uk/evidence-based-veterinary-medicine/ebvm-resources/clinical-trials (accessed 6 January 2022).

Russell, W.M.S. and Burch, R.L. (1959). The principles of humane experimental technique. http://117.239.25.194:7000/jspui/bitstream/123456789/1342/1/PRILIMINERY%20%20AND%20%20CONTENTS.pdf.

RVC (2021). VetCompass. www.rvc.ac.uk/vetcompass (accessed 21 March 2021).

Select Statistical Services (2021). Calculators. https://select-statistics.co.uk/calculators (accessed 8 May 2021).

Siedlecki, S.L. and Albert, N.M. (2017). Research-active clinical nurses: against all odds. *J. Clin. Nurs.* 26: 766–773. https://doi.org/10.1111/jocn.13523.

Studer, A and Abbott, B. (2020). SUBJECT GUIDES – Evidence-Based Practice Resources. https://www.library.ucdavis.edu/guide/ebp-resources (accessed 9 March 2021).

The Caldicott Committee (1997). Report on the Review of Patient-Identifiable Information. https://webarchive.nationalarchives.gov.uk/20130124064947/www.dh.gov.uk/prod_consum_dh/groups/dh_digitalassets/@dh/@en/documents/digitalasset/dh_4068404.pdf (accessed 18 March 2021).

University of Nottingham (2021). BestBETS for Vets. https://bestbetsforvets.org (accessed: 9 March 2021).

VetAUDIT (2021). The National Audit for Small Animal Neutering (NASAN). https://vetaudit.rcvsk.org/nasan (accessed 20 March 2021).

Viner, B. (2009). Using audit to improve clinical effectiveness. *In Pract.* 31: 240–243.

Wainc, K. and Brennan, M. (2015). Clinical audit in veterinary practice: theory v reality. *In Pract.* 37: 545–549. http://doi.org/10.1136/inp.h5457.

Wylie, C.E. (2015). Prospective, retrospective or clinical audit: a label that sticks. *Equine Vet. J.* 47: 257–259.

Index

Page locators in **bold** indicate tables. Page locators in *italics* indicate figures. This index uses letter-by-letter alphabetization.

Professionalism and Reflection in Veterinary Nursing, First Edition.
Edited by Sue Badger and Andrea Jeffery.
© 2022 John Wiley & Sons Ltd. Published 2022 by John Wiley & Sons Ltd.
Companion website: www.wiley.com/go/badger/professionalism-veterinary-nursing